GET THROUGH

MRCP: PACES

Dedication

We would like to dedicate this book to our families, for their unconditional and unprecedented love. We would also like to thank our friends for their loyalty and support.

GET THROUGH

MRCP: PACES

Rajeev Gulati - BSc MBBS MRCP DRCOG MRCGP AHEA
GP Principal, London; FY2 supervisor, London and Eastern Deaneries

Monal Wadhera - BSc MBBS MRCP DRCOG MRCGP DFSRH AHEA MA
GP Principal, London; GP tutor, London Deanery;
NIHR In Practice Fellow

Edited by Iñaki Bovill - BSc MBBS FRCP
Consultant Physician and Geriatrician, Chelsea and Westminster Hospital

Foreword by Eric Beck - Former Chairman of the MRCP (UK) Part 2 Board and Former Chairman of the PACES Implementation Committee

CRC Press
Taylor & Francis Group
Boca Raton London New York

CRC Press is an imprint of the
Taylor & Francis Group, an informa business

CRC Press
Taylor & Francis Group
6000 Broken Sound Parkway NW, Suite 300
Boca Raton, FL 33487-2742

First issued in hardback 2017

Version Date: 20130226

ISBN-13: 978-1-85315-834-6 (pbk)
ISBN-13: 978-1-138-45120-9 (hbk)

Visit the Taylor & Francis Web site at
http://www.taylorandfrancis.com

and the CRC Press Web site at
http://www.crcpress.com

CONTENTS

FOREWORD

Assessment drives learning! This was the mantra that underpinned the major restructuring of all parts of the MRCP(UK) examination in the 1990s, resulting in the replacement of the Oral, Long and Short Cases by PACES (Practical Assessment of Clinical Examination Skills). Leading up to this was a lengthy process of learning, observation and consultation involving other evolving medical examinations and the burgeoning new academic discipline of Medical Education, culminating in convening an international conference. I had the privilege of being part of this exciting project.

A syllabus of the knowledge and skills required by a trainee specialist in General (Internal) Medicine was drawn up. This acted as a template to ensure which different parts of the examination would best cover most of the syllabus requirements.

Reproducibility between worldwide examination centres and from one examination to another required standardization of content and marking against pre-agreed criteria by trained examiners whose training would be regularly updated. (A very few traditionalist and individualist examiners fell by the wayside.) Detailed check-list type mark sheets, customized for each station, 'drive' the five PACES stations, recording detailed performance data to give feedback to the unsuccessful candidate. The long-established and tested principles of the undergraduate OSCE (Objective Structured Clinical Examination), pioneered in Dundee, have been adapted to a postgraduate setting.

Needless to say a 'cottage industry' of courses and books has developed to familiarize candidates with the 'new' MRCP and help them prepare for it. The authors of this book are obviously 'battle hardened' and streetwise from their own successful study and preparation. The contents are up to date and certainly have authenticity. There is much practical advice on the knowledge required and how to best present it under examination conditions. They frequently remind the reader/candidate to supplement the book with individual study and of the prerequisite of practising with like-minded colleagues and willing mentors.

I commend it to readers and wish them the final ingredient for success – good luck!

Eric Beck
Former Chairman of the MRCP(UK) Part 2 Board and Former Chairman of the PACES Implementation Committee

ABOUT THE AUTHORS

Dr Rajeev Gulati qualified from university college London in 2000 with a BSc in Psychology. He achieved a Certificate of Merit for outstanding performance as well as Certificate of Merit in Clinical Pharmacology in MBBS written finals. He successfully completed the MRCP in 2003 at his first attempt. He worked as a medical registrar and then completed a year as an emergency registrar in Sydney, Australia. Rajeev subsequently backpacked around Southeast Asia. Thereafter, he moved into general practice and completed the MRCGP exams.

Rajeev currently works as a full time GP partner in North London and has an active role within medical education. He is an FY2 supervisor and is actively involved in teaching medical students and other trainees within the practice. He is currently undertaking the Teaching the Teacher (TTT) course to become a GP trainer. He completed the Certificate in Learning and Teaching (CILT) at QMUL in 2010 and is an Associate Member of the Higher Education Academy. He is an examiner for medical students at Kings College London medical school and has written books for both the MRCP and MRCGP examinations. His interests include running, travel and playing with his baby girl.

Dr Monal Wadhera qualified from Imperial College at St Mary's in 2002 with a BSc in Cardiovascular Medicine. She successfully completed the MRCP in 2005 on her first sitting. She subsequently decided on a career in General Practice. She trained on the West Middlesex Vocational Training Scheme and qualified in 2007, achieving the MRCGP with distinction. She was awarded the 'Great Expectations' Bursary by the Royal College of General Practitioners in 2007.

Monal is a GP Principal in London and has a keen interest in medical education, having completed the MA in Clinical Education at the Institute of Education. She holds posts as GP Tutor with the London Deanery and Clinical Lead in Professional Development at Hammersmith & Fulham Primary Care Trust. She was awarded the National Institute for Health Research In-Practice Fellowship by the Department of Health in 2010. She achieved a distinction in the Certificate in Learning and Teaching at Queen Mary University of London and merit in the Royal College of General Practitioners Leadership Programme. She is an examiner for medical students at Queen Mary University of London and has written previous revision guides for the MRCP and MRCGP examination. She is also a GP appraiser, which she enjoys greatly. Outside medicine, her interests include dining, reading, travelling, writing and yoga.

Dr Iñaki Bovill qualified from Charing Cross and Westminster Medical School in 1993 and subsequently trained as a General Physician Geriatrician in the North West Thames region including at St Mary's Hospital and Chelsea & Westminster

Hospital. He was appointed to the consultant staff at Chelsea & Westminster Hospital in 2004 where he has developed an interest in peri-operative medicine providing support to the General Surgeons and Orthopaedic teams (including pre-operative optimization), Rehabilitation Medicine supporting the Rehabilitation Unit at Ellesmere House and continence. His clinical interests also include all aspects of Elderly and General Medicine but particularly the complex elderly patient and polypharmacy.

ACKNOWLEDGEMENTS

We are extremely grateful to so many people without whose help this book would not have been possible. Firstly, we would like to acknowledge Dr Iñaki Bovill, Consultant Geriatrician at Chelsea and Westminster Hospital, who has spent much time and energy editing this book. Iñaki has been a fabulous mentor, particularly when he led our team as Consultant Geriatrician. He is now both a good friend and a colleague who has always taken great pride in his work and maintained the highest of standards. We are also very grateful to Eric Beck for writing the Foreword for this book. Clearly, Eric Beck has made an enormous contribution towards the PACES exams. We would like to thank the following for their invaluable contributions towards the photographs in this book: Dr Begoña Bovill, MSc, MRCP, DTM&H; Dr Aruna Dias, Consultant Gastroenterologist; Dr Omar Malik, Consultant Neurologist; Mr Eoin O'Sullivan, Consultant Ophthalmologist; Shamira Perera, MBBS (Hons), BSc (Hons), FRCOphth; Mr Hiten G. Sheth, Consultant Opthalmologist; Dr Sandeep Panikker, Bsc, MBBS, MRCP, SPR in Cardiology and Electrophysiology Research Fellow; and Mr Wai Weng Yoon, BSc (Hons), MBBS, FRCS Tra & Orth, Senior Clinical Lecturer, RNOH Stanmore. A big thank you to Abha Gulati for helping with research for the book. Gabar Singh, Jai and Veeru were great sources of inspiration during the writing of this book.

We would like to thank the National Institute for Health and Clinical Excellence for allowing us to use their material. Finally, we would like to thank the Royal Society of Medicine and Sarah Penny, Stephen Clausard and the team at Hodder Arnold for their patience and support throughout the process of preparing this book.

ABBREVIATIONS

ABPA	Allergic bronchopulmonary aspergillosis
ACE	Angiotensin-converting enzyme
ACTH	Adrenocorticotrophic hormone
ADH	Antidiuretic hormone
ADPKD	Adult polycystic kidney disease
A&E	Accident and emergency (department)
AF	Atrial fibrillation
AFP	α-fetoprotein
AIDS	Acquired immune deficiency syndrome
AIH	Autoimmune hepatitis
ALL	Acute lymphocytic leukaemia
ALP	Alkaline phosphatase
ALT	Alanine transaminase
AMA	Anti-mitochondrial antibody
AML	Acute myeloid leukaemia
ANA	Antinuclear antibody
AR	Aortic regurgitation
ARB	Angiotensin receptor blocker
ARMD	Age-related macular degeneration
ASD	Atrial septal defect
ASO	Anti-streptolysin O
AST	Aspartate transaminase
BCC	Basal cell carcinoma
BCG	Bacille Calmette–Guérin
b.d.	Bis in die (twice daily)
BIPAP	Bilevel positive airway pressure
BMI	Body mass index
BP	Blood pressure
CCF	Congestive cardiac failure
CF	Cystic fibrosis
CFP	Culture filtrate protein
CFTR	Cystic fibrosis transmembrane regulator
CJD	Creutzfeldt–Jakob disease
CK	Creatine kinase
CLL	Chronic lymphocytic leukaemia
CML	Chronic myeloid leukaemia
CMV	Cytomegalovirus
CN	Cranial nerve
CNS	Central nervous system
COMT	Catechol-O-methyltransferase
COPD	Chronic obstructive pulmonary disease
COX	Cyclo-oxygenase
CPA	Cerebellopontine angle
CPK	Creatine phosphokinase
CREST (syndrome)	Calcinosis, Raynaud's phenomenon, oesophageal dysmotility, sclerodactyly and telangiectasia
CRP	C-reactive protein
CRT	Cardiac resynchronization therapy
CSF	Cerebrospinal fluid
CT	Computed tomography
CVA	Cerebrovascular accident

CXR	Chest radiograph
DMARD	Disease-modifying antirheumatic drug
DNA	Deoxyribonucleic acid
DNR	Do not resuscitate (order)
DPP-4	Dipeptidyl peptidase 4
DVLA	Driver and Vehicle Licensing Agency
DVT	Deep vein thrombosis
EAA	Extrinsic allergic alveolitis
EBV	Epstein–Barr virus
ECG	Electrocardiography
ELISPOT	Enzyme-linked immunosorbent spot assay
EMG	Electromyography
ENT	Ear, nose and throat
ERCP	Endoscopic retrograde chloangiopancreato-graphy
ESAT	Early secretory antigen target
ESR	Erythrocyte sedimentation rate
FBC	Full blood count
FBG	Fasting blood glucose
FEV_1	Forced expiratory volume
FSH	Follicle-stimulating hormone
FVC	Forced vital capacity
FY1, FY2	Foundation year 1, foundation year 2
GGT	γ-glutamyl transpeptidase
GH	Growth hormone
GLP-1	Glucagon-like peptide 1
GN	Glomerulonephritis
GORD	Gastro-oesophageal reflux disease
GTN	Glyceryl trinitrate
GTT	Glucose tolerance test
HGPRT (deficiency)	Hypoxanthine–guanine phosphoribosyltrans-ferase (deficiency)
HIV	Human immunodeficiency virus
HLA	Human leucocyte antigen
HOCM	Hypertrophic obstructive cardiomyopathy
HSP	Henoch – Schonleih purpura
HSV	Herpes simplex virus
HTLV-1	Human T-cell lymphotrophic virus type I
IBD	Inflammatory bowel disease
IBS	Irritable bowel syndrome
ICD	Implantable cardiovertes–defibrillator
ICU	Intensive care unit
Ig	Immunoglobulin
IGF-1	Insulin-like growth factor
IPJ	Interphalangeal joint
IPPV	Intermittent positive pressure ventilation
ITP	Idiopathic thrombocytopaenic purpura
IV	Intravenous
IVC	Inferior vena cava
IVU	Intravenous urography
JCVI	Joint Committee on Vaccination and Immunisation
JVP	Jugular venous pressure
LDH	Lactate dehydrogenase
LDL	Low-density lipoprotein
LFT	Liver function test
LH	Luteinizing hormone
LMN	Lower motor neuron
LP	Lumbar puncture
LTOT	Long-term oxygen therapy
LVEF	Left ventricular ejection fraction
LVF	Left ventricular failure
LVH	Left ventricular hypertrophy

MAOI	Monoamine oxidase inhibitor
MCPJ	Metacarpophalangeal joint
MCV	Mean cell volume
MEN	Multiple endocrine neoplasia
MI	Myocardial infarction
MND	Motor neuron disease
MPTP	1-methyl-4-phenyl-1,2,3,6-tetradydropyridine
MRI	Magnetic resonance imaging
MS	Multiple sclerosis
MSH	Melanocyte-stimulating hormone
MSU	Mid-stream urine
MTPJ	Metatarsophalangeal joint
NICE	National Institute for Health and Clinical Excellence
NSAID	Non-steroidal anti-inflammatory drug
o.d.	Omni in die (every day)
OGTT	Oral glucose tolerance test
$Paco_2$	Partial pressure of carbon dioxide in arterial blood
Pao_2	Partial pressure of oxygen in arterial blood
PAN	Polyarteritis nodosa
p-ANCA	Perinuclear anti-neutrophil cytoplasmic antibody
PBC	Primary bilary cirrhosis
PD	Parkinson's disease
PDA	Patent ductus arteriosus
PE	Pulmonary embolus
PET	Positron emission tomography
PID	Pelvic inflammatory disease
PIPJ	Proximal interphalangeal joint
PMR	Polymyalgia rheumatica
PND	Paroxysmal nocturnal dyspnoea
PNS	Peripheral nervous system
p.r.n.	Pro re nata (when required)
PRV	Polycythaemia rubra vera
PSA	Prostate-specific antigen
PSC	Primary sclerosing cholangitis
PT	Prothrombin time
PTH	Parathyroid hormone
PUVA	Psoralen combined with ultraviolet A
q.d.s	Quater die sumendus (to be taken four times daily)
RA	Rheumatoid arthritis
RAPD	Relative afferent pupillary defect
RF	Rheumatoid factor
RNA	Ribonucleic acid
RVF	Right ventricular failure
RVH	Right ventricular hypertrophy
SACD	Subacute combined degeneration of the cord
SCC	Squamous cell carcinoma
SIADH	Syndrome of inappropriate anti-diuretic hormone excess
SLE	Systemic lupus erythematosus
SRP	Signal recognition particle
STI	Sexually transmitted infection
SVC	Superior vena cava
SVCO	Superior vena cava obstruction

SVT	Supraventricular tachycardia
TB	Tuberculosis
t.d.s	Ter die sumendum (to be taken three times daily)
TEN	Toxic epidermolysis necrosis
TFT	Thyroid function test
TIA	Transient ischaemic attack
TIBC	Total iron-binding capacity
TIPJ	Terminal inter-phalangeal joint
TIPS	Transjugular intrahepatic portosystemic shunt
TLC	Total lung capacity
TNF–α	Tumour necrosis factor
TOE	Transoesophageal echocardiography
TPHA	*Treponema pallidum* haemagglutination assay
TRH	Thyroid-releasing hormone
TSH	Thyroid-stimulating hormone
U&E	Urea and electrolytes
UMN	Upper motor neurone
USS	Ultrasound scan
UTI	Urinary tract infection
UVB	Ultraviolet B
VATS	Video-assisted thoracoscopic surgery
VDRL	Venereal Disease Research Laboratory
VSD	Ventricular septal defect
VT	Ventricular tachycardia
VTE	Venous thromboembolism
WCC	White cell count
WHO	World Health Organization

INTRODUCTION

We have written this book as an aid to preparation for the MRCP PACES (Practical Assessment of Clinical Examination Skills) examination.

We have structured the book into the format of the exam, such that each chapter represents a station. We have included cases that commonly present in MRCP PACES exams.

We have also included a chapter on examination skills, which outlines how to examine each system.

The cases in this book are laid out as in the exam setting. They begin with scenario information typical of what you will receive in the exam. The structuring of the information provided for each case follows the format you will encounter in the exam. In each case discussion, we have followed a question and answer style to mimic a conversation with the examiner. This format allows you to recreate realistic scenarios for all the stations. This approach is useful in private study and for role-playing with colleagues. This can be used to practise with colleagues or on your own, and we found this a very useful approach to adopt when revising for the PACES exam ourselves.

We have included photographs throughout the book to give a useful overall impression of selected conditions. There is also a chapter of supplementary cases at the back of the book with a collection of photographs, including many on eye and skin conditions. These could arise in a variety of contexts throughout the exam, so they have been placed in a separate chapter where they are easily accessible. They include many conditions that are often used as spot diagnoses and therefore may be used to test yourself in private study or in groups. Alongside each photo we have included useful clinical information structured as possible question and answer scenarios.

Although we have included a wide breadth of scenarios and discussion points, please remember that the content of this book is not exhaustive, and it is important to read around any topics you come across that are not included here. The further reading recommendations are sources of information that will also be useful in preparing for the exam.

About the MRCP PACES exam and preparation tips

PACES exam format

The MRCP PACES exam is the clinical part of the MRCP(UK) Part 2 exam. It can be taken before or after the MRCP(UK) Part 2 written exam as long as both Part 2 exams are taken within 7 years of passing the MRCP (UK) Part 1 written exam.

The PACES exam is structured into five clinical stations as shown below.

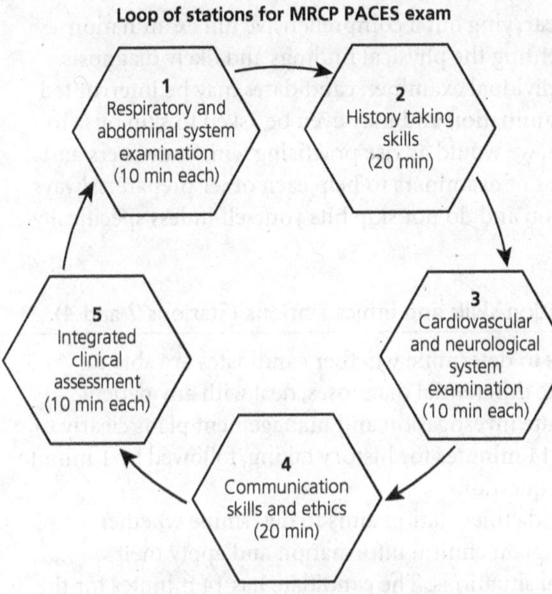

The five clinical stations in the MRCP PACES exam.

Station 1 – Respiratory (10 minutes) and abdominal (10 minutes) system examination
Station 2 – History taking (20 minutes)
Station 3 – Cardiovascular (10 minutes) and neurological (10 minutes) system examination
Station 4 – Communication skills and ethics (20 minutes)
Station 5 – Two brief clinical consultations (10 minutes each)
Each candidate passes through five clinical stations, each of which last 20 minutes each, in a clockwise fashion, and there is a 5-minute break between stations.

Exam details and tips

The PACES exam aims to test the following seven skills:

- Physical examination
- Identifying physical signs
- Communication skills
- Differential diagnosis
- Clinical judgement
- Handling patient concerns
- Ensuring patient welfare

Examination stations (Stations 1 and 3)

The examination stations aim to determine whether candidates are able to perform correct examination techniques, identify physical signs, generate differential diagnoses and suggest appropriate investigation and management plans. The candidate has 6 minutes for each examination followed by 4 minutes of questions.

Candidates should practise carrying out a comprehensive full examination within the 6 minutes and presenting the physical findings and likely diagnosis. However, depending on the individual examiner, candidates may be interrupted with questions during their examination and may even be asked to skip bits. To avoid this becoming a problem, we would advise practising with your peers and taking the role of different types of examiners to help each other prepare. Always assume a structured examination and do not skip bits yourself unless specifically asked to do so.

History taking and communication skills and ethics stations (Stations 2 and 4)

The history taking station aims to determine whether candidates are able to adequately gather data, generate differential diagnoses, deal with any patient concerns and suggest appropriate investigation and management plans clearly to the patient. The candidate has 14 minutes for history taking, followed by 1 minute for reflection and 5 minutes of questions.

The communication skills and ethics station aims to determine whether candidates are able to clearly explain clinical information and apply their knowledge and ethics to clinical situations. The candidate has 14 minutes for the interview, followed by 1 minute for reflection and 5 minutes of questions. The scenario at this station will often involve a complex situation, which is associated with a difficult ethical dilemma, or sensitive situations.

For Stations 2 and 4, the written scenario is given to the candidate to read during the 5-minute interval. We found that this was a good opportunity to note the main points you wish to cover during the scenario. This acts as an aide-memoire, which will assist you when under pressure.

A good way to approach these stations is to adopt good verbal and non-verbal skills and use a mixture of open and closed questions. Following up on cues is also essential as this may lead you to important information.

Brief clinical consultation station (Station 5)

The brief clinical consultation station aims to determine whether candidates are able to approach a focused clinical scenario, encompassing a targeted history, examination and communication. The candidate has 8 minutes for each scenario followed by 2 minutes to describe the physical signs and differential diagnoses.

Throughout all of the stations, it is important to treat the patient with dignity and respect.

Patients

Each of the clinical stations (1, 3 and 5) will have real patients present, whereas the history taking and communication skills and ethics stations (2 and 4) tend to have actors playing the role of a patient.

Examiners

Each station has two examiners, each marking candidates separately without conferring. There is a different set of examiners for each station, giving a total of 10 examiners for the whole exam.

Marking scheme

There are structured mark sheets for each station (two for each of the examination and brief consultation stations and one for each of the history taking and communications stations). As there are two examiners at each station, there will be a total of 16 marksheets. These are given to candidates at the beginning of the exam for them to fill out their personal details (name, examination number and centre number). The mark sheets are then handed to the relevant examiners at each station.

Candidates are marked as **Satisfactory, Borderline** or **Unsatisfactory** on each of the seven defined skills listed above, which will be variably tested at each station. Each grade reflects a numerical value between 0 and 2 (unsatisfactory = 0; borderline = 1; satisfactory = 2). The MRCP(UK) board sets the pass marks for each of the seven skills and for the whole exam annually in advance. In order to pass the PACES exam, candidates need to achieve *both* the minimum marks for each skill *and* the minimum marks for the whole exam.

Borderline or Unsatisfactory results have to be accompanied by explanatory comments that can then be used to give feedback to failing candidates.

Sample mark sheets for each station and details of the pass marks are available on the MRCP(UK) website (www.mrcpuk.org/PACES/Pages/).

Results

Results are made available on the MRCP(UK) website approximately 10 days after the exam.

In cases of a 'fail', candidates are able to retake the PACES exam an unlimited number of times as long as it is within 7 years of passing the MRCP(UK) Part 1 exam.

Preparation for the exam

Go to www.mrcpuk.org/PACES/Pages/ for information about the PACES exam. The website has up-to-date details about applying for the exam, required conduct at the exam, preparation for the day and getting your results. There are also sample scenarios and mark sheets, which are well worth looking at.

Our overall advice in preparing for the exam is simple: practise, practise, practise!

Practicing on patients

It is best to practise with colleagues or show an interest during ward rounds with your senior colleagues and encourage them to viva you. The scenarios you will see in these circumstances are likely to come up in some form. Practise on patients until the examination routines are familiar and then read around the subjects using this book.

Familiarizing yourself with the techniques under pressure

Another way to practise is when seeing patients in the accident and emergency (A&E) or outpatient department. This is a good opportunity to take a history or consider the communications and ethics around various scenarios. Discuss cases with your colleagues and read around the subjects as you go along. Remember, unlike the Part I and Part II written exams, this is a practical exam.

Exam conditions

Try to recreate exam conditions by working in pairs or small groups in which each person takes it in turns to be examined or carry out the role of examiner. Be strict with time limits and follow the marking schemes for feedback.

PACES courses

We would recommend doing a PACES course. Besides putting yourself into the exam situation, it also provides the opportunity to see patients with less common clinical conditions that you may not have seen on the wards.

Location

PACES exams are carried out at various centres around the country. Often candidates have to travel long distances and stay overnight. It is important to plan ahead, ensure that you know where the exam is and, if possible, rehearse the walk to the hospital. Hospital departments can be difficult to find at the best of times.

On the day

Ensure that you set out to arrive early in case there are delays. Examiners can pick up on a candidate who is stressed and tired. It is therefore important to arrive at the exam well rested and as relaxed as possible.

PART I

PRACTICE EXAM STATIONS

1 STATION 1 RESPIRATORY AND ABDOMINAL SYSTEM

RESPIRATORY SYSTEM

Pulmonary fibrosis

Describe your clinical findings

On examination, this patient is short of breath at rest with a respiratory rate of 18 breaths/minute. She has rheumatoid arthritis of the hands, as evidenced by wasting of the small muscles of the hands, ulnar deviation and deformity of the fingers. Her fingers are also clubbed and she is cyanosed. There are several purpura on the arms suggestive of steroid use. Chest expansion is reduced. On auscultation of the chest there are bilateral, fine inspiratory crackles at both lung bases.

These findings suggest a diagnosis of pulmonary lung fibrosis. In view of the rheumatoid hands, the likely underlying diagnosis is rheumatoid disease.

TOP TIPS

- Look for other signs of autoimmune disease, rash such as butterfly rash of SLE or changes in hands and face associated with systemic sclerosis.
- Look for cushingoid features arising from the use of steroids.

What do you understand by the term pulmonary fibrosis?

This condition occurs when there is abnormal and excessive deposition of fibrotic tissue in the lung parenchyma, resulting in impaired gas transfer.

What are the causes of interstitial lung disease?

- Cryptogenic fibrosing alveolitis
- Connective tissue disease:
  - rheumatoid lung disease
  - systemic sclerosis
  - SLE
  - polymyositis
  - dermatomyositis

  - Sjögren's syndrome
  - mixed connective tissue disease
- Ankylosing spondylitis
- Sarcoidosis
- Asbestosis
- Silicosis
- Extrinsic allergic alveolitis
- Radiation
- Drugs such as bleomycin, nitrofurantoin and amiodarone

What are the causes of upper lobe fibrosis?

Remember: BREADTHS

- **B**eryliosis
- **R**adiation, when the upper lobe is not shielded
- **E**xtrinsic allergic alveolitis
- **A**nkylosing spondylosis
- **A**llergic bronchopulmonary aspergillosis
- **D**rugs
- **T**uberculosis
- **H**istiocytosis X
- **S**ilicosis
- **S**arcoidosis

What are the causes of lower lobe fibrosis?

Remember: SCRAD

- **S**cleroderma
- **C**ryptogenic fibrosing alveolitis
- **R**heumatoid arthritis
- **R**adiation, when the lower lobe is not shielded
- **A**sbestosis
- **D**rugs

With what symptoms and signs do patients with pulmonary fibrosis present?

- Shortness of breath
- Non-productive cough
- Clubbing
- Malaise
- Weight loss
- Cyanosis
- Fine bilateral inspiratory crackles
- Signs of associated disease

What drugs are linked to pulmonary fibrosis?

- Methotrexate
- Cyclophosphamide

- Amiodarone
- Gold
- Nitrofurantoin
- Sulfonamides

How would you investigate this patient?

Blood tests

- ESR – raised
- RF and ANA – can be positive
- Hypergammaglobulinaemia
- Arterial blood gases – to assess the degree of hypoxia

Imaging

- CXR shows bilateral basal reticulonodular changes.
- High-resolution CT scan shows 'honeycombing'.

Other tests

- Lung function tests:
  - restrictive pattern: $FEV_1/FVC > 0.8$
  - reduced diffusion capacity (K_{co})
- Broncho-alveolar lavage:
  - lymphocytes suggest a good prognosis and good response to steroids
  - neutrophils suggest a poor prognosis and poor response to steroids
- Lung biopsy may be needed

How would you manage this condition?

- Smoking cessation if the patient is a smoker
- Avoid environmental causes
- Stop any medications thought to cause pulmonary fibrosis
- Provide the patient with influenza and pneumococcal vaccination
- Immunosuppressant drugs such as steroids, cyclophosphamide and azathioprine
- Lung transplantation if disease progresses and the patient is fit for surgery
- Long-term oxygen therapy for patients with significant hypoxia

What are the pulmonary manifestations of rheumatoid disease?

- Interstitial lung disease
- Pleural effusion
- Pulmonary arteritis
- Pulmonary nodules
- Obliterative bronchiolitis

What tests on pleural fluid in a patient with a pleural effusion suggest rheumatoid disease?

- RF +ve
- Exudate (high in protein)

- Raised LDL
- Low glucose
- Reduced C3 and C4
- WCC < 5000/μL

What are the complications of pulmonary nodules in patients with rheumatoid disease?

- The nodules have a predilection for the upper lobes
- They often resemble cancer and tuberculosis
- Complications include:
  - haemoptysis
  - pleural effusion
  - bronchopulmonary fistulas
  - can become infected and cavitate
  - can rupture into the pleural space leading to a pneumothorax

What do you know about Caplan's syndrome?

- This is the combination of pulmonary nodules in rheumatoid disease and coal worker's pneumoconiosis (due to mining dust).
- Lung function tests show a mixed restrictive and obstructive picture.
- Patients are treated with steroids.

What do you know about extrinsic allergic alveolitis (EAA)?

- In this condition, there is a hypersensitivity reaction affecting the lung parenchyma causing diffuse, granulomatous inflammation in response to repeated inhalation of organic antigens in dust.
- Patients can present acutely, sub-acutely or with chronic respiratory problems.
- Acute presentations are usually due to Type III (immune complex-mediated) hypersensitivity reactions causing a pneumonitis.
- Chronic presentations are usually due to Type IV (cell mediated) hypersensitivity reactions and lead to fibrosis.
- Several antigens are responsible but the provoking antigen in an individual can be difficult to identify.
- EAA can be associated with many occupations and hobbies as seen in the table below.

Table 1 Classification and causes of EAA

Name	Antigen
Bird fancier's lung	Avian proteins in bird feathers and faeces
Farmer's lung	Mouldy hay containing *Saaccharopolyspora rectivirgula*
Cheese-worker's lung	Mouldy cheese containing *Penicillum casei*
Malt-worker's lung	Mouldy malt containing *Aspergillus clavatus*
Mushroom-worker's lung	Mushroom compost containing thermophilic actinomycetes
Chemical-worker's lung	Trimellitic anhydride, diisocyanate and methylene diisocyanate found in plastics, polyurethane foam and rubber manufacturing
Hot-tub lung	*Mycobacterium avium* found in poorly maintained hot tubs

How do patients with EAA present?

(a) Acute presentation

- Symptoms start 4–8 hours after exposure to the antigen and resolve within days.
- The duration and severity of symptoms are related to the level of exposure. Low-level acute exposure may produce mild symptoms for only a few hours. In very severe cases, patients may develop life-threatening respiratory failure with cyanosis, respiratory distress and high fever.
- Symptoms include:
  - flu-like illness with fever
  - dry cough
  - shortness of breath
  - chest tightness
  - anorexia
  - malaise
  - headache
  - generalized aches and pains
- Signs include:
  - fever
  - tachypnoea
  - bilateral basal fine inspiratory crackles.

(b) Sub-acute presentation

- Patients who present sub-acutely may have a history of repeated acute attacks.
- Symptoms tend to be gradual and less severe, although severe life-threatening episodes can occur.
- After the exposure is removed, it can take weeks or months for symptoms to resolve.
- Symptoms include:
  - cough
  - shortness of breath
  - fatigue
  - anorexia
  - weight loss
  - recurrent pneumonia
- Signs are as for acute presentation.

(c) Chronic presentation

- Patients with chronic disease usually have permanent lung damage. Removal of the antigen may have minimal improvement on symptoms.
- Symptoms include:
  - weight loss
  - worsening shortness of breath
- Signs include:
  - cyanosis
  - clubbing

  - tachypnoea
  - bilateral basal inspiratory crackles
- Chronic hypoxia leads to pulmonary hypertension with right heart failure.

What blood test would you request, in addition to those listed above for pulmonary fibrosis?

- Serum antibodies or precipitans may be detectable e.g. IgG antibody to pigeon gammaglobulin but many have no detectable antibodies.
- Inflammatory makers may be raised but this is non-specific.

What other tests may you undertake?

- CXR: can be normal or show reticular opacities in upper fields in the acute or sub-acute forms. Upper lung fibrosis with loss of lung volume is seen in chronic disease.
- High resolution CT.
- Lung function tests reveal a restrictive defect.
- Bronchoalveolar lavage reveals lymphocytosis and the CD4/CD8 ratio is <1.
- Lung biopsy may be needed and shows the characteristic histopathological features.

How do you manage patients with EAA?

- Avoidance of allergen exposure is important in patients with acute and chronic EAA. Allergen avoidance usually results in recovery for patients presenting with acute EAA. This nlay require a change in occupation.
- LTOT to treat hypoxaemia.
- Corticosteroids may be indicated for severe acute and subacute presentations as well as for chronic forms. However, steriods do not alter the long-term outcome.

What do you know about asbestos and lung disease?

- Asbestos exposure can affect people working in ship building, lagging, construction workers and those working in factories in which asbestos products are manufactured.
- Asbestos exposure can cause a wide range of lung disease such as:
  - pleural plaques
  - diffuse pleural thickening
  - pleural effusions
  - asbestosis
  - increased risk of lung cancer and mesothelioma

Asbestos and the lung

Pleural plaques

- Appear ~20 years after asbestos exposure.
- Usually asymptomatic but can cause mild restrictive lung disease.
- Can develop on the pleura, diaphragm, mediastinum and pericardium.

Diffuse pleural thickening

- Mainly affects the lung bases.
- Causes exertional dyspnoea.
- Lung function tests show restrictive lung disease with reduced total lung capacity.

Asbestosis

- Appears ~20 years after asbestos exposure.
- Fibrosis occurs mainly in the lower lobes.
- Patients can present with exertional dyspnoea.
- Examination reveals clubbing and fine inspiratory crackles.
- Lung function tests show restrictive lung disease and reduced gas transfer.
- There is an increased risk of lung cancer and mesothelioma.
- Patients are entitled to industrial compensation.

Mesothelioma

- Develops from mesothelial cells in the pleura or, less commonly, the peritoneum.
- Asbestos is responsible for the vast majority of malignant mesotheliomas.
- Crocidolite (blue asbestos) is the most toxic, followed by amosite (brown asbestos) and then cryosolite (white asbestos) which is the least toxic.
- There is a latent period, usually ~30 or more years, between asbestos exposure and mesothelioma development.
- Patients can present with chest pain, shortness of breath, dry cough or weight loss.
- Diagnosis is made by pleural biopsy.
- Treatment is with surgery and radiotherapy.
- Patients are eligible for industrial compensation.

Lung cancer

- The risk of lung cancer is increased 5-fold.
- The combination of asbestos and smoking increases the risk of cancer 55-fold.

Name some other occupational lung diseases

Table 2 Occupational Lung Diseases

Name	Caused by Exposure to
Silicosis	Silicon dioxide
Berylliosis	Beryllium
Byssinosis	Cotton dust, flax and hemp
Coal worker's pneumoconiosis	Mining dust

Bronchiectasis

Describe your clinical findings

On examination, this patient is cachectic and tachypnoeic, with a respiratory rate of 18 breaths/minute. He has bilateral clubbing of the fingers and cyanosis. The sputum pot contains copious amounts of green-coloured sputum. On auscultation of the chest, there are left (or right) crepitations in the lower zones and widespread wheeze.

These findings suggest a diagnosis of bronchiectasis.

What is bronchiectasis?

This is a chronic infection of the bronchi and bronchioles leading to abnormal, permanent dilation of the airways.

What are the causes of bronchiectasis?

- Bronchial obstruction due to bronchial tumour, external compression from lymphadenopathy or inhalation of a foreign body
- Respiratory infection in childhood (measles, pertussis and tuberculosis)
- Cystic fibrosis
- Marfan's syndrome
- Kartagener's syndrome
- Hypogammaglobulinaemia
- Allergic bronchopulmonary aspergillosis (ABPA)

How do you investigate patients with bronchiectasis?

Tests to confirm bronchiectasis

- Sputum culture and cytology
- Chest radiograph (CXR) shows tramlines and ring shadows (thickened bronchial walls)
- High-resolution computed tomography (CT) scan shows thickened, dilated bronchi that are larger than the adjacent vascular bundles ('signet' sign)

Tests to determine the underlying cause

- Bloods to check immunoglobulin levels and detect hypogammaglobulinaemia
- Skin prick test for *Aspergillus* to check for aspergillosis precipitins
- Sweat test to detect cystic fibrosis (CF)
- Electron microscopy of cilia from nasal or tracheal mucosa to check for Kartagener's syndrome
- Bronchoscopy to exclude malignancy or foreign body

What are the common pathogens that cause infections in bronchiectasis?

- *Haemophilus influenzae*
- *Staphylococcus aureus*
- *Pseudomonas aeruginosa*

How do you manage patients with bronchiectasis?

- Physiotherapy to aid postural drainage
- Antibiotics for short-term exacerbations; long-term antibiotics may be needed

- Bronchodilators to help airflow obstruction
- Inhaled or oral steroids may be helpful in certain cases
- Surgery with lobe resection can be curative in patients with localized disease

List some complications of bronchiectasis

- Pneumonia
- Empyema
- Pleural effusion
- Cor pulmonale
- Haemoptysis
- Amyloidosis
- Cerebral abscess due to haematogenous spread of infection

What are the features of Kartagener's syndrome?

- Kartagener's syndrome is an autosomal recessive condition where the primary defect is in the structure and function of cilia. Features include:
  - bronchiectasis
  - dextrocardia
  - situs invertus
  - infertility
  - sinusitis
  - otitis media
  - dysplasia of the frontal sinuses

Cystic fibrosis

Describe your clinical findings

On examination this young patient appears underweight. He is tachypnoeic with a respiratory rate of 18 breaths/minute. He has bilateral clubbing of his fingers and a productive cough. The sputum pot contains a large amount of green sputum. Chest expansion is reduced. On auscultation of the chest, there are crepitations over the lower zones of the left (± right) lung. There is a widespread polyphonic expiratory wheeze.

These findings suggest the patient has bronchiectasis. In a young patient, the likely diagnosis is CF.

What do you know about CF?

- Autosomal recessive disorder affecting 1 in 2500 Caucasians.
- 1 in 20 are carriers.
- Most cases are due to a mutation at position 508 on chromosome 7, which results in a deletion of phenylalanine. The chloride channel, CF transmembrane regulator (CFTR), is defective and chloride secretion from cells is therefore reduced.
- As a result, exocrine secretions have a high concentration of sodium and a low concentration of chloride and water. The secretions are thickened and viscid and so block the lumens of ducts and organs, such as the gut.

What are the clinical features of the disease?

Respiratory

- Nasal polyps
- Haemoptysis
- Recurrent chest infections
- Bronchiectasis
- Sinusitis
- Respiratory failure
- Pneumothorax
- Pulmonary fibrosis
- Cor pulmonale
- ABPA

Gastrointestinal

- Rectal prolapse
- Meconium ileus
- Steatorrhoea
- Pancreatitis
- Gallstones
- Biliary cirrhosis
- Liver cirrhosis and portal hypertension resulting from biliary strictures

Other

- Arthropathy
- Diabetes
- Infertility in males
- Sub-fertility in females
- Failure to thrive

What investigations would you perform?

- Heel prick test at birth showing raised level of immunoreactive trypsin
- Sweat sodium test shows sodium > 60 mmol/L
- Genetic testing

Name some pathogens that cause acute exacerbations in patients with CF

- *Staphylococcus aureus*
- *Haemophilus influenzae*
- *Pseudomonas aeruginosa*
- *Burkholderia cepacia*

How do you manage patients with CF?

- Physiotherapy to aid postural drainage and breathing techniques
- Antibiotics – can be oral, nebulized or IV
- Bronchodilators for symptomatic relief

- Pancreatic supplements to reduce the risk of malabsorption
- Recombinant human DNAse, which degrades DNA in the bronchial secretions
- Immunizations for measles, influenza and pneumococcus
- Heart and lung transplant
- Gene therapy
- Genetic counselling for couples

Pleural effusion

Describe your clinical findings

On examination this patient is comfortable at rest. His respiratory rate is 12 breaths/minute. Chest expansion is reduced on the left side and the percussion note is stony dull at the left base. On auscultation of the chest, vocal resonance and breath sounds are reduced. There is an area of bronchial breathing above the area of the dullness.

These findings are suggestive of a pleural effusion.

What are the other cases of dullness at a lung base?

- Pleural effusion
- Collapse
- Consolidation
- Pleural thickening
- Raised hemi-diaphragm (can occur with hepatomegaly)

What are the causes of pleural effusion?

Exudates (protein > 30 g/L)	Transudates (protein < 30 g/L)
• Lung malignancy (primary or secondary)	• Cardiac failure
• Mesothelioma	• Nephrotic syndrome
• Pneumonia	• Liver cirrhosis
• Tuberculosis	• Meigs' syndrome
• Pulmonary embolus	• Hypothyroidism
• Rheumatoid arthritis	
• SLE	
• Lymphoma	

What is Meigs' syndrome?

- This is a right-sided pleural effusion due to an ovarian fibroma.

What drugs can cause a pleural effusion?

- Methysergide
- Methotrexate
- Nitrofurantoin

How would you investigate this patient?

- Pleurocentesis
- Pleural biopsy
- CXR (anterior–posterior and lateral)
- CT scan of thorax to confirm pleural effusion
- Bronchoscopy if malignancy considered

What tests would you do on the pleural fluid?

Biochemistry

- Protein concentration: > 30 g/L suggests an exudate and < 30 g/L suggests a transudate.
- LDH is raised in empyema, malignancy, TB, RA and SLE.
- Amylase is raised in pancreatitis, malignancy and pneumonia.
- Glucose is reduced in empyema, malignancy, TB, RA and SLE.
- RF or ANA may be positive in pleural fluid in autoimmune conditions.

Microbiology and culture

- Gram or Ziehl–Neelsen stain

Cytology

- Malignant cells may be present in neoplastic conditions.
- Red blood cells suggest malignancy, pulmonary infarction or TB.
- Neutrophils are raised in effusions arising from pneumonia.
- Lymphocytes are raised in infection, malignancy, autoimmune conditions and TB.
- Eosinophils are raised in pneumothorax and asbestos-related effusions.

What are Light's criteria?

An exudate is considered present when:

- The ratio of pleural fluid albumin to the plasma albumin > 0.5.
- The ratio of pleural fluid LDH to the plasma LDH > 0.6.
- The pleural fluid LDH is > two-thirds of the normal level of plasma LDH.

Pneumonectomy and lobectomy

Describe your clinical findings

Pneumonectomy

On examination, this patient is comfortable at rest. There is a thoracotomy scar on the left chest wall, which is flattened. The trachea and apex beat are deviated to the left side. Chest expansion is reduced on the left (affected) side and the percussion note is dull. On auscultation of the chest, the breath sounds are reduced.

These findings suggest a left-sided pneumonectomy.

Lobectomy

On examination this patient is comfortable at rest. There is a thoracotomy scar on the left chest wall, which is flattened. The trachea is central and the apex beat is not displaced. Chest expansion is normal but the percussion note is dull in the left lower zone. On auscultation of the chest, the breath sounds are reduced.

These findings suggest a left-sided lobectomy.

What are the indications for pneumonectomy or lobectomy?

- Carcinoma
- Pulmonary nodules
- Bronchiectasis
- TB – before chemotherapy was available

Chronic obstructive pulmonary disease (COPD)

Describe your clinical findings

On examination this patient is short of breath at rest (may have oxygen cylinder) with a respiratory rate of 18 breaths/minute. The fingers have nicotine stains, but there is no carbon dioxide retention flap of the hands. He is cyanosed and his lips are pursing during expiration. He has a plethoric appearance and is using his accessory muscles of respiration. The chest is hyperinflated and chest expansion is normal. There is a tracheal tug. The percussion note is resonant. On auscultation of the chest, the breath sounds are reduced and have a prolonged expiratory phase. There is widespread expiratory wheeze.

These findings suggest a diagnosis of COPD due to cigarette smoking.

What is COPD?

- COPD is a term encompassing the spectrum of disease from chronic bronchitis to emphysema. It is a chronic, progressive disease.
- Chronic bronchitis is a clinical diagnosis. It is defined as a cough productive of sputum on most days for more than 3 months of 2 consecutive years in the absence of other diseases causing sputum production.
- Emphysema is a pathological diagnosis. There is permanent enlargement of the airway distal to the respiratory bronchioles with the destruction of alveolar walls.

What are the causes of emphysema?

- Smoking is the commonest cause.
- Industrial dust exposure (coal dust in mine workers or cadmium exposure) can cause emphysema.
- α1-antitrypsin deficiency is rare but should be considered in a young patient who does not smoke.

What is α_1-antitrypsin deficiency?

- α_1-antitrypsin is a protease inhibitor enzyme which inhibits neutrophil elastase. It is primarily synthesized in the liver.
- The condition results from mutations of the gene on chromosome 14.
- There are a few genetic variants – M for normal, S for slow and Z for very slow.
- Deficiency of α_1-antitrypsin means that neutrophil elastase in the lungs is no longer inhibited. This leads to excessive breakdown of the alveolar walls.
- Patients develop basal, pan-lobular emphysema and liver cirrhosis.

What investigations would you perform?

- Bloods to check for:
  - elevated white cells (acute infection)
  - low levels of α_1-antitrypsin
  - polycythaemia may be present
- Sputum culture
- CXR shows hyperinflated lungs and bullae. Complications of COPD such as pneumothorax may be found
- Arterial blood gas to assess the degree of hypoxia
- Spirometry shows an obstructive pattern:
  - $FEV_1/FVC < 70\%$
  - $FEV_1 < 80\%$

How do you manage patients with COPD?

- Please refer to NICE guidance (2010) Chronic obstructive pulmonary disease. NICE Guideline CG 101. London: NICE.

Medical management

- Smoking cessation is the single most beneficial management strategy
- Bronchodilators
- Inhaled steroids if COPD is steroid responsive
- Aminophylline
- Long-term oxygen therapy (LTOT)
- Vaccinations – influenza annually and pneumococcal every 5–10 years
- Pulmonary rehabilitation including exercise, smoking cessation, nutritional assessment and education about the disease

Surgical management

- Bullectomy
- Lung reduction surgery
- Lung transplant

What are the criteria for LTOT?

- Non-smoker
- $FEV_1 < 1.5$ L
- $FVC < 2$ L

- Pao_2 < 7.3 kPa on air or 7.3–8.0 kPa if there is pulmonary hypertension or nocturnal hypoxia
- $Paco_2$ that does not rise excessively with oxygen treatment
- Evidence of cor pulmonale

How do you treat patients with an acute exacerbation of COPD?

- 24% oxygen via a Venturi mask
- Nebulized bronchodilators
- Oral or intravenous antibiotics (depending on severity)
- Oral steroids; consider IV hydrocortisone in severe cases
- IV aminophylline
- Non-invasive ventilation with BIPAP in severe cases where the patient is tiring and $Paco_2$ is rising
- IPPV if good pre-morbid quality of life

What treatment can you use for patients to help the symptoms of shortness of breath?

- Promethazine
- Dihydrocodeine

Lung malignancy

Describe your clinical findings

Case 1

On examination, this patient appears cachectic. The fingers are stained with nicotine and are clubbed. There is a lymph node in the left supraclavicular fossa. The trachea is deviated to the left (same side as the lesion) and chest expansion is reduced on the left. The percussion note is dull at the left base. On auscultation of the chest, vocal resonance is increased over the area of dullness while breath sounds are reduced.

These clinical findings suggest left basal consolidation, probably due to malignancy.

Case 2

On examination, this patient's fingers are stained with nicotine and are clubbed. There is a lymph node in the left supraclavicular fossa. The trachea is deviated to the right (away from the lesion) and chest expansion is equal. The percussion note is stony dull at the left base. On auscultation of the chest, vocal resonance and breath sounds are reduced over the area of dullness.

These clinical findings suggest a left-sided pleural effusion, probably due to malignancy.

Case 3

On examination, the fingers of this patient are stained with nicotine and are clubbed. There is wasting of the small muscles of the left hand, with reduced sensation in the T1 dermatome. There is a left Horner's syndrome and axillary lymphadenopathy. The trachea is central and chest expansion is equal. On auscultation of the chest, vocal resonance and breath sounds are reduced at the left apex of the chest.

These clinical findings suggest the presence of a left-sided Pancoast's tumour.

TOP TIPS

- Look for lobectomy scars or radiotherapy burns or tattoos.
- Look for complications of lung malignancy such as SVCO, dermatomyositis and acanthosis nigricans.

What are the types of lung cancer?

- Small cell lung cancer (25%)
- Non-small cell lung cancer (75%):
  - squamous cell
  - adenocarcinoma
  - large cell

What are the risk factors associated with lung cancer?

- Smoking
- Air pollution
- Pulmonary fibrosis
- Occupational exposure to asbestos, silicon, arsenic and cadmium

How do patients with lung cancer present?

- Cough
- Weight loss
- Haemoptysis
- Shortness of breath
- Recurrent chest infections
- Hoarseness of the voice (left-sided lesions cause recurrent laryngeal nerve palsy)
- Horner's syndrome
- SVCO
- Paraneoplastic syndromes (see below)
- Symptoms relating to metastatic spread (see below)

Where does lung cancer spread to?

- Brain
- Liver
- Bone
- Adrenal glands

What is the definition of a paraneoplastic syndrome?

These syndromes are a consequence of a cancer in the body. These phenomena are mediated by humoral factors (hormones or cytokines) excreted by tumour cells or by an immune response against the tumour.

Which paraneoplastic syndromes are associated with lung cancer?

Endocrine

- Gynaecomastia
- PTH-related peptide secretion by squamous cell tumours causing hypercalcaemia
- Cushing's syndrome due to ectopic ACTH secretion by small cell tumours
- SIADH due to ectopic ADH secretion by small cell tumours
- Carcinoid syndrome due to carcinoid tumours

Neurological

- Lambert–Eaton syndrome
- Paraneoplastic cerebellar degeneration

Skin

- Dermatomyositis
- Acanthosis nigricans

What are the complications of carcinoma of the bronchus?

Respiratory

- Cough
- Chest pain
- Haemoptysis
- Dyspnoea
- Stridor
- Rib erosion
- Pleural effusion
- Recurrent chest infections
- Bronchiectasis
- Lung abscess
- Lobar collapse
- SVCO

Endocrine

- Gynaecomastia
- SIADH
- PTH-related peptide secretion
- ACTH secretion causing Cushing's syndrome

Neurological

- Brachial plexus invasion
- Metastases

- Peripheral neuropathy
- Polymyositis
- Lambert–Eaton syndrome
- Proximal myopathy
- Cerebellar degeneration

Cardiovascular

- Anaemia
- Atrial fibrillation
- DVT
- Non-bacterial thrombotic endocarditis

Skin

- Dermatomyositis
- Acanthosis nigricans
- Erythema gyratum migrans

Other

- Horner's syndrome
- Recurrent laryngeal nerve palsy
- Hypertrophic pulmonary osteoarthropathy

How do you investigate patients with lung cancer?

- Sputum cytology
- Bloods to check liver function tests, calcium, sodium and haemoglobin
- CXR to confirm the presence of a mass
- Pleural fluid aspiration
- CT scan of thorax to stage the disease
- Bone scan to check for metastases to the bone
- PET scan
- Bronchoscopy – for histological diagnosis
- Lung function tests to assess whether suitable for surgery

How do you treat patients with lung cancer?

Small cell tumours

- Chemotherapy
- Usually disseminated and rarely operable

Non-SCC

- Surgery – lobectomy or pneumonectomy
- Radiotherapy
- Chemotherapy

Palliative care

- Pain is managed with opiates and radiotherapy.
- Pleural effusions can be managed with chemical pleurodesis.
- SVCO can be treated with dexamethasone and radiotherapy.
- Brain metastases can be treated with dexamethasone and radiotherapy.

What are the indications for radiotherapy?

- Pain
- Haemoptysis
- Bronchial obstruction
- SVCO
- Pancoast's tumour

Old tuberculosis

Describe your clinical findings

Case 1

On examination, this patient is comfortable at rest. There is a left-sided upper chest deformity. The trachea is deviated to the left side (same side as the fibrosis/thoracotomy scar). Chest wall expansion is reduced on the left upper chest wall and the percussion note at the left apex is dull. On auscultation of the chest, bronchial breathing and crepitations are present at the left apex. There is a posterior thoracotomy scar where some of the ribs have been resected (Figure 1).

These findings suggest that the patient has had a thoracotomy for the treatment of TB.

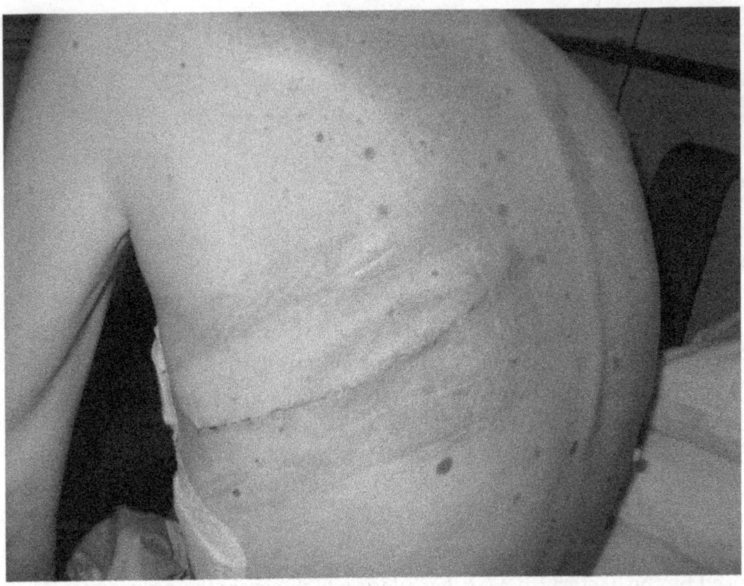

Figure 1 Left lateral thoracotomy scar. Reproduced with permission of Sandeep Panikker.

Case 2

On examination, this patient is comfortable at rest. There is a left supraclavicular scar. Chest expansion is reduced on the left side. The percussion note is dull at the left base. On auscultation, there are reduced (or absent) breath sounds at the left lung base.

The patient has had a phrenic nerve crush for the treatment of tuberculosis.

Case 3

On examination, this patient is comfortable at rest. The trachea is deviated to the left side (same side as the fibrosis). Chest wall expansion is reduced on the left upper chest wall and the percussion note at the left apex is dull. On auscultation of the chest, bronchial breathing and crepitations are present at the left apex.

This patient has left-sided apical pulmonary fibrosis, most likely due to old TB.

How was TB treated prior to the days of chemotherapy?

- TB was treated by inducing apical lung collapse. It was thought that this would deprive the causative agent, *Mycobacterium tuberculosis*, of oxygen and so prevent its proliferation.
- Techniques used were:
  - rest and sunbathing
  - artificial pneumothorax to collapse the diseased area of the lung
  - plombage which involved insertion of polystyrene balls into the thoracic cavity
  - thoracoplasty which involved the removal of ribs
  - phrenic nerve crush which involved the paralysis of the diaphragm leading to diminished movements of the lung on the side of the paralysis

What are the complications of old TB?

- Bronchiectasis
- Pleural effusion
- Aspergillomas can develop in the old TB cavity
- Scarring from TB predisposes to bronchial carcinoma

Tuberculosis

Describe your clinical findings

On examination, this patient is comfortable at rest. His respiratory rate is 12 breaths/minute. Chest expansion is normal and equal on both sides. The trachea is central. The percussion note is dull at the left apex. On auscultation, there is increased vocal resonance with crepitations and bronchial breathing over the left apex.

These findings suggest that the patient has left apical consolidation. The differential diagnosis includes TB, bronchial carcinoma, pneumonia or pulmonary infarction.

Tell me about TB

- This is caused by the bacterium *M. tuberculosis* which enters the pulmonary system by droplet spread.

- It is a notifiable disease.
- TB is common in Asia and Eastern Europe. Rates in the UK are increasing.
- It is a granulomatous inflammatory condition.
- The pathogenesis of TB can be described in terms of primary, post-primary and miliary tuberculosis.

Primary TB

- The tubercle bacillus is initially inhaled, causing primary pulmonary TB.
- It may occasionally infect the tonsils or gastrointestinal tract.
- Infection in the lung results in the development of a 'primary complex', which is a combination of the primary (Ghon) focus of the infection in the lung tissue and the development of caseous hilar lymphadenopathy.
- Patients are usually asymptomatic although they may develop:
  - persistent cough
  - fever
  - erythema nodosum
  - lung collapse due to compression on the bronchus
- In the majority of patients, the primary complex heals and calcifies. Spread is prevented by the regional lymph nodes.
- In a minority of patients, the primary infection develops into post-primary TB.
- The tuberculin test is positive 4–8 weeks after primary tuberculosis.

Post-primary TB

- This usually results from reactivation of an old lesion but can occur due to direct progression of a primary lesion that fails to heal.
- Post-primary TB can affect the lung (post-primary pulmonary TB) or spread to various organs haematogenously (see below).

Systemic symptoms

- Anorexia
- Night sweats
- Fever
- Weight loss

Post-primary pulmonary

- Cough
- Pneumonia
- Aspergilloma
- Haemoptysis
- Empyema
- Pleural effusion

Pott's disease

- TB of the spine causing abscess and vertebral collapse

Genitourinary tuberculosis

- Dysuria
- Haematuria
- PID
- Loin pain
- Sterile pyuria
- Infertility

Meningeal tuberculosis

- TB meningitis
- Cerebral tuberculomas

Tuberculous peritonitis

- Ascites
- Abdominal pain

Skin

- Erythema nodosum
- Lupus vulgaris

Tuberculous pericarditis

- Pericardial effusion
- Constrictive pericarditis

Tuberculous lymphadenitis

- Cold abscesses
- Painless lymphadenopathy

Gastrointestinal tuberculosis

- Diarrhoea
- Obstruction
- Malabsorption

Adrenal tuberculosis

- Adrenal insufficiency

Miliary TB

- This is characterized by widespread dissemination of bacteria to various organs, including the lungs, leading to multiple foci.
- It has a characteristic appearance on CXR.

What factors lead to reactivation of an old lesion?

This is due to any form of immunosuppression:

- Malnutrition
- Alcoholism
- Cigarette smoking
- Immunosuppressant drugs such as steroids
- Silicosis and other occupational disease
- Diseases with impaired cellular immunity:
  - HIV or AIDS
  - Hodgkin's disease
  - leukaemia
  - lymphoma

Which groups of people are at high risk of contracting TB?

- Asian immigrants
- Alcoholics
- Contacts of known TB cases
- The elderly
- Immunocompromised individuals
- Healthcare workers – doctors, nurses, carers

How do you diagnose patients with TB?

Tuberculin skin test

- Heaf test is used as a screening test
- Mantoux test:
  - >10 mm at 72 hours is considered positive
  - suggests immunity from BCG vaccination, previous exposure or may indicate active infection if strongly positive

Chest radiograph

- Cavitation
- Upper lobe consolidation

Microbiology

- Test sputum with Ziehl–Neelsen staining
- Pleural aspiration or biopsy
- Early MSU
- Bone marrow biopsy
- Lymph node biopsy
- Bronchial lavage
- Gastric washings
- CSF examination

Immunological testing with interferon-γ release assays

- This has replaced Heaf/Mantoux testing in many centres.
- *M. tuberculosis* produces antigens:
  - early secretory antigen target 6 (ESAT-6) and
  - culture filtrate protein 10 (CFP-10)
- These antigens stimulate host production of interferon-γ.
- These tests are useful as the antigens are not present in non-tuberculous mycobacterium or any BCG vaccine variant and so help to distinguish latent TB infection.
- Lymphocytes from the patient's blood are incubated with TB antigens.
- The QuantiFERON test measures the *production of interferon-γ* that is released from T-lymphocytes that have been incubated with TB antigens.
- The TB ELISPOT (enzyme-linked immunosorbent spot assay) measures the *number of activated T-lymphocytes* that secrete interferon-γ.

How do you treat patients with tuberculosis?

- Standard treatment regimens usually last for 6 months, but 12 months will be required if the patient has tuberculous meningitis.

Before treatment

- Stress the importance of compliance.
- Check baseline liver and renal function.
- Consider an HIV test.
- Assess colour vision before and during treatment (ethambutol can cause ocular toxicity).

Drug treatment

Antibiotics

- Start treatment before the culture results are available if symptoms and signs suggest tuberculosis.
- Standard regimen:
  - 2 months of four-drug therapy: isoniazid, rifampicin, pyrazinamide, ethambutol
  - 4 months of two-drug therapy: isoniazid and rifampicin
- Pyridoxine is given to prevent neuropathy related to isoniazid.

Steroids

- These may be needed in tuberculous meningitis and pericarditis.

Note

Drug resistance to TB is increasing, especially in patients who are HIV positive or have AIDS and so antibiotic treatment may need to alter once cultures are available.

Name some of the side effects of these drugs

Isoniazid

- Hepatitis
- Neuropathy

Rifampicin

- Hepatitis
- Inactivates contraceptive pill
- Orange discolouration of the urine

Pyrazinamide

- Hepatitis
- Arthralgia

Ethambutol

- Optic neuritis – colour vision is affected first

What do you know about the BCG vaccination?

- The BCG vaccine is a live attenuated strain of *Mycobacterium tuberculosis* which confers a degree of immunity in some individuals.
- BCG vaccination confers up to 80% protection for up to 15 years. It does not guarantee protection against TB.
- It is more effective in children than in adults.
- The Joint Committee on Vaccination and Immunisation (JCVI) has recommended that the following risk groups be offered BCG vaccination in the UK:
  - all infants living in areas where the incidence of TB is 40/100 000 or greater
  - infants whose parents or grandparents were born in a country with a TB incidence of 40/100 000 or greater
  - children who would otherwise have been offered BCG through the schools' programme (this was administration of the BCG vaccine to all previously unvaccinated children aged 10–14 years) will be screened for risk factors, tested and vaccinated as appropriate
  - contacts of known cases
  - those at risk due to their occupation (healthcare workers, veterinary staff, prison staff)
  - previously unvaccinated new immigrants from countries with a high prevalence of TB
  - those intending to live or work in high-prevalence countries for extended periods (generally 1 month or longer)

Lung transplant

Describe your clinical findings

Case I

On examination, this patient is comfortable at rest. His respiratory rate is 14 breaths/minute. He has bilateral clubbing of the fingers. There is a mid-sternotomy scar. Chest expansion and percussion note are normal. On auscultation of the chest, there are normal vesicular breath sounds.

These findings, together with a history of chest infections, suggest that the patient has had a double lung transplantation for CF.

Case 2

On examination, this patient is comfortable at rest. She has a respiratory rate of 14 breaths/minute. She has bilateral clubbing of the fingers and rheumatoid arthritis of the hands. She has several purpura, suggestive of steroid treatment, on both arms. She has a right thoracotomy scar. Chest expansion is equal and the percussion note is dull at the left base. On auscultation of the chest, there are fine inspiratory crackles in the lower zone of the left lung.

This patient has had a right lung transplant for the treatment of pulmonary fibrosis which has probably arisen as a consequence of rheumatoid disease. She appears to be on steroid therapy.

What are the indications for lung transplantation?

- COPD
- Bronchiectasis
- CF
- Pulmonary fibrosis
- α_1-antitrypsin deficiency
- Primary or secondary pulmonary hypertension

In what circumstances would a lung transplant be contraindicated?

- Alcoholism
- Smoking
- HIV
- Hepatitis
- Chronic illness such as kidney or liver disease

What are the types of lung transplant?

- Lobe
- Single lung
- Double lung
- Heart–lung

What are the complications of lung transplantation?

- Rejection (hyperacute, acute or chronic):
  - chronic rejection can result in bronchiolitis obliterans
  - occurs months to years after a lung transplant
  - characterized by fibrosis and scarring of the small airways
  - symptoms include persistent cough, shortness of breath and fatigue
  - lung function tests show worsening airflow obstruction, reduced TLC and gas transfer
  - immunosuppressants often fail and re-transplantation is needed
- Infections including bacterial, viral (CMV, HSV) and fungal (*Candida*, *Aspergillus* spp.)
- Side effects of immunosuppressant drugs such as steroids, azathioprine and ciclosporin
- Re-development of original disease
- Malignancy, particularly skin cancers and lymphomas

Chest consolidation

Describe your clinical findings

On examination, this patient is short of breath with a respiratory rate of 18 breaths/minute. He is on 2 L of oxygen via nasal cannulae. The sputum pot contains some green sputum. The trachea is central. Chest wall expansion is reduced on the left side and the percussion note over the left base is dull. On auscultation of the chest, there is an increase in vocal resonance over the left base, bronchial breathing and coarse crepitations.

These findings suggest left basal consolidation. I would like to check the temperature chart to see if the patient has a fever. This would suggest the patient has pneumonia.

TOP TIP

- Clubbing may indicate empyema.
- Erythema multiforme indicates *Mycoplasma* infections.

What are the causes of consolidation?

- Pneumonia
- Carcinoma
- Pulmonary embolus
- Pulmonary vasculitis

How would you investigate this patient?

- Blood tests to check WCC, CRP, urea, liver function tests and atypical serology
- Blood cultures
- Sputum cultures and microscopy
- Arterial blood gas to check for hypoxia
- CXR to confirm consolidation
- Urine to check for *Legionella* antigen

What are the common pathogens leading to community-acquired pneumonia?

- *Streptococcus pneumoniae*
- *H. influenzae*
- *Mycoplasma pneumoniae*
- *Chlamydia pneumoniae*
- *Legionella* spp.
- Influenza A and B

How do you treat community-acquired pneumonia?

- Amoxicillin 500 mg t.d.s. for 7 days orally *or*
- Add in erythromycin 500 mg q.d.s. if atypical pneumonia suspected
- Give erythromycin 500 mg q.d.s. if allergic to penicillin *or*
- Clarithromycin 500 mg b.d. (twice daily) if intolerant to erythromycin *or*
- IV cephalosporin plus macrolide if the infection is severe

What are the common pathogens leading to hospital acquired pneumonia?

- *Pseudomonas* spp.
- *Staphylococcus aureus*
- Other gram-negative bacilli such as *Klebsiella*

How do you treat hospital acquired pneumonia?

- IV cephalosporin ± gentamicin

What are the complications of pneumonia?

- Lung abscess
- Pleural effusion
- Pneumothorax
- Septicaemia
- Respiratory failure

What is the CURB-65 score?

- This measures the severity of community-acquired pneumonia.
- It helps to define the need for hospital admission and guides treatment (e.g. IV as opposed to oral antibiotics):
  - **C**onfusion
  - **U**rea > 7 mmol/L
  - **R**espiratory rate > 30 per minute
  - **BP** systolic < 90 mmHg or diastolic < 60 mmHg
  - **65** years or older

Table 3 Assessing risk with the CURB – score

Score	Management	Risk of death at 30 days
0	Can be managed as an outpatient	0–0.6%
1	Can be managed as an outpatient	3.2%
2	Can be managed as an outpatient with close monitoring but may need to be admitted	13.0%
3	Admit to hospital	17%
4	Admit to hospital	41.5%
5	Admit to hospital	57%

What do you know about the extrapulmonary features of *Mycoplasma pneumoniae?*

Extrapulmonary features

- Otitis media
- Pericarditis
- Myocarditis

- Erythema multiforme
- Erythema nodosum
- Haemolytic anaemia
- Meningioencephalitis
- Transverse myelitis
- Cranial and peripheral neuropathies
- Hepatitis
- Pancreatitis
- Steven–Johnson syndrome

Treatment

- Macrolide (erythromycin or clarithromycin) or tetracycline.

What do you know about the extrapulmonary features of *Legionella pneumoniae?*

Extrapulmonary features

- Diarrhoea
- Jaundice
- Ileus
- Pancreatitis
- SIADH
- Acute renal failure

Treatment

- Macrolide (erythromycin or clarithromycin)
- Rifampicin may be added in severe infections

Superior vena cava obstruction (SVCO)

On examination this patient is comfortable at rest. The face appears plethoric and suffused. The upper limbs are oedematous. The superficial veins on the chest wall are dilated and the neck veins are engorged and non-pulsatile. There is a radiation burn on the chest wall.

These findings suggest a diagnosis of SVCO, which is being treated by radiotherapy.

What are the causes?

- Carcinoma of the bronchus
- Lymphoma
- Thymoma
- Mediastinal tumour
- Thoracic aortic aneurysm
- Mediastinal fibrosis
- Mediastinal goitre

What are the clinical features?

- Headaches
- Dysphasia
- Dizziness
- Blackouts
- Shortness of breath and stridor

What are the treatment options?

- Radiotherapy
- Chemotherapy
- Dexamethasone
- Stent insertion to the SVC

Pneumothorax

Describe your clinical findings

On examination, this patient is tall and thin. He is comfortable at rest with a respiratory rate of 12 breaths/minute. Chest expansion on the left side is reduced. Percussion note on the left side is hyper-resonant. On auscultation of the chest, vocal resonance and breath sounds are reduced.

These findings suggest a diagnosis of a left-sided pneumothorax. I would like to confirm the diagnosis with a CXR.

How do you manage patients with a pneumothorax?

Treatment depends on the severity of the pneumothorax:

- Small – spontaneously resolve in weeks
- Larger – simple aspiration
  - chest drain for 24 hours
  - remove if the lung has expanded
  - if the lung has not re-expanded, use suction
- Pleurodesis can be used for recurrent pneumothoraces.

What are the indications for a chest drain?

- Large pneumothorax
- Tension pneumothorax
- Pneumothorax complicating underlying severe chronic bronchitis with emphysema
- Pneumothorax exacerbating underlying asthma

How do you manage a tension pneumothorax?

- Released urgently by inserting an IV cannula in the second intercostal space, mid-clavicular line

How do you manage patients with recurrent pneumothoraces?

- Pleurodesis is a procedure used to obliterate the pleural space permanently by attaching the lung to the chest wall. It prevents recurrence of pneumothorax and pleural effusion.
- Pleurodesis can be performed surgically or chemically.

- Surgical pleurodesis can be performed via thoracotomy or thoracosopy through video-assisted thoracoscopic surgery (VATS). These procedures involve pleurectomy (removal of the outer pleura) and pleural abrasion (mechanically irritating the inner pleura). During the healing process, the inner pleura and lung adhere to the chest wall, thus obliterating the pleural space.
- VATS reduces hospital admission and post-operative pain, and is associated with fewer complications than thoracotomy.
- Chemical pleurodesis involves the use of chemicals such as talcum powder or antibiotics such as bleomycin or tetracycline. The agents are passed into the lung through a chest tube or during VATS. These substances activate an inflammatory process that causes the lung to adhere to the chest wall. However, the results are worse than for the surgical procedures.

What are the causes of pneumothorax?

- Spontaneous
- Trauma
- COPD
- Asthma
- Pneumonia
- Carcinoma of the lung
- TB
- CF
- Mechanical ventilation
- Rheumatoid lung disease
- Marfan's syndrome
- Sarcoidosis
- Histiocytosis X

ABDOMINAL SYSTEM

Jaundice

Describe your clinical findings

This patient is jaundiced. He has several other peripheral features of chronic liver disease such as .... On examination of the abdomen there is hepatomegaly, with the liver being enlarged ... cm below the right costal margin.

I would like to finish my examination by checking the urine.

How would you define jaundice?

Jaundice is the yellowish discolouration of the skin, sclera and mucous membranes due to hyperbilirubinaemia.

How is bilirubin produced?

- Bilirubin is the end product of haem metabolism.
- 80% of bilirubin is produced from the breakdown of haem from haemoglobin in red blood cells and 20% from the breakdown of haem in myoglobin and cytochromes.

What causes jaundice?

Pre-hepatic causes

- Jaundice occurs when bilirubin is increased through exercise, haemoglobin breakdown (haemolysis) or myoglobin breakdown (rhabdomyolysis).
- Haemolysis can be intrinsic (where the RBC is defective) or extrinsic (where the RBC is normal).

Intrinsic Causes	*Extrinsic Causes*
• Disorders of RBC membrane • Hereditary – spherocytosis – elliptocytosis • Acquired – paroxysmal nocturnal haemoglobinuria (PNH)	• Immune • Haemolytic disease of the newborn • Blood transfusion incompatibility • Autoimmune haemolytic anaemia
• Disorders of Hb synthesis • Sickle-cell anaemia • Thalassaemia • Deficiencies of RBC enzymes • Glucose-6-phosphatase deficiency • Pyruvate kinase deficiency	• Non-immune • Prosthetic valves • Hypersplenism • Infections e.g. malaria

Rhabdomyolysis

Causes of rhabdomyolysis include:

- Muscle trauma:
  - crush injury
  - falls and prolonged immobility
  - burns
  - polymyositis
- Drugs and toxins:
  - statins
  - alcohol
- Infections:
  - septicaemia
  - viral, e.g. coxsackie virus and EBV

Hepatic causes

- Bilirubin increases in any process in which cell necrosis reduces the liver's ability to metabolize and excrete bilirubin such as:
  - acute hepatitis and liver cirrhosis of any cause
  - enzymopathies such as Gilbert's syndrome and Crigler–Najjar syndrome

Post-hepatic causes

- Bilirubin levels increase when there is an obstruction in the biliary drainage system causing the build up of bile products.
- Obstruction can occur within the liver or outside it:

Intrahepatic	*Extrahepatic*
PBC	Gallstones
PSC	Pancreatic carcinoma
Drugs	Parasites

Table 4 Investigations in jaundice

Parameter	Pre-hepatic	Hepatic	Post-hepatic
Bilirubin	↑	↑	↑
Conjugated bilirubin	N	N/↓	↑
Unconjugated bilirubin	↑	↑	N
Urobilinogen	↑	↑	↓
Colour of urine	N	Dark	Dark
Colour of stool	N	N	Pale
Aspartate transaminase (AST)/Alanine transaminase (ALT)	N	↑	Normal
Alkaline phosphatrase (ALP)	N	N	↑
Reticulocyte count	↑	N	N
Haptoglobulins	↓	N	N

How would you investigate patients with jaundice?

Blood tests

- FBC
- LFTs
- Haptoglobulins
- Reticulocyte count
- Coombs' test
- Clotting studies
- Autoimmune screen
- Viral screen

Urine tests

- Urine for bilirubin and urobilinogen

Further tests

- USS of abdomen
- CT scan of abdomen
- ERCP
- Liver biopsy

What is Gilbert's syndrome?

- It is an autosomal dominant condition resulting in reduced levels of the enzyme glucuronyltransferase. This results in reduced conjugation of bilirubin.
- Levels of unconjugated bilirubin are increased.
- It is precipitated by stress, fasting or infection.
- The condition is benign and patients are asymptomatic.
- No further treatment is necessary.

What is Dubin–Johnson syndrome?

- It is an autosomal recessive defect of molecular transporters responsible for excreting conjugated bilirubin out of hepatic cells.
- It leads to increased levels of conjugated bilirubin and pigmentation of the liver.

Chronic liver disease

Describe your clinical findings

Hands

- Clubbing
- Leuconychia
- Hyperpigmentation
- Excoriation
- Purpura
- Xanthomata
- Dupytren's contracture
- Palmar erythema
- Hepatic flap

Abdomen

- Hepatomegaly
- Splenomegaly
- Hepatosplenomegaly
- Ascites
- Caput medusa

Chest

- Spider naevi
- Gynaecomastia

Face

- Jaundice

Other features

- Scanty body hair
- Testicular atrophy
- Ankle oedema
- Tattoos
- Needle marks suggesting intravenous drug use

Mention some of the causes of liver disease

- Alcohol abuse
- Viral hepatitis (hepatitis B or C)
- Autoimmune chronic active hepatitis
- PBC
- Metabolic disorders – haemochromatosis, Wilson's disease, α_1-antitrypsin deficiency
- Drugs – methyldopa, amiodarone, methotrexate
- Cardiac failure
- Budd–Chiari syndrome
- Biliary obstruction
- Cryptogenic

What investigations would you carry out?

Bloods

- LFTs
- GGT
- Iron
- Ferritin
- FBC
- Autoantibody screen
- Clotting
- AFP
- Hepatitis B and C screen
- Caeruloplasmin

Analysis of ascitic fluid

- Determine whether an exudate or transudate
- Microscopy (WCC seen in spontaneous bacterial peritonitis) and culture

Liver biopsy

Imaging

- USS of liver and biliary tract

What is the definition of cirrhosis?

- Cirrhosis is a consequence of chronic liver disease.
- It is characterized by a replacement of normal liver tissue by fibrous scar tissue and regenerative nodules, which leads to a loss of liver function.

What are the complications of liver cirrhosis?

- Ascites
- Spontaneous bacterial peritonitis
- Coagulopathy
- Portal hypertension
- Variceal haemorrhages
- Hepatic encephalopathy
- Hepatorenal syndrome
- Hepatocellular carcinoma

What can precipitate hepatic encephalopathy?

- Infection
- Drugs: diuretics and sedatives
- Upper gastrointestinal haemorrhage
- Abdominal paracentesis
- Surgery

Tell me about AIH

- Affects females more than males.

- Associated with autoimmune conditions such as diabetes, thyroiditis, RA, scleroderma and inflammatory bowel disease.
- Presents with fatigue, right upper quadrant pain, arthralgia and abnormal LFTs.
- Treatment is with immunosuppressive drugs such as steroids and azathioprine.

Classification of AIH

Type I

- Accounts for 80% of AIH.
- Associated with HLA B8/DRw3, ANA, anti-smooth muscle antibodies and polyclonal hypergammaglobulinaemia.

Type II

- Accounts for 10% of AIH.
- Associated with anti-liver/kidney/microsomal antibodies.
- Not associated with ANA.

Type III

- Rapidly progressive and associated with anti-soluble liver antigen antibodies.

Tell me about α_1-antitrypsin deficiency

- Caused by defective production of α_1-antitrypsin, which is a protease inhibitor.
- There are several forms and degrees of deficiency.
- Deficiency results in cirrhosis and increased risk of hepatocellular carcinoma.
- Severe deficiency causes pulmonary emphysema in adult life.
- Treatment is by liver and lung transplantation.
- See also p.16.

Tell me about hepatitis B

- It is a DNA virus.
- Transmitted parenterally or by sexual contact.
- Complications include liver cirrhosis and hepatocellular carcinoma.
- Treatment with interferon-α is successful in about 40% of cases.
- Side effects include flu-like symptoms, depression, fatigue and haematological abnormalities.
- Other drug treatments include lamivudine, adefovir and entecavir.

Tell me about hepatitis C

- It is an RNA virus.
- The main routes of transmission are through needles in intravenous drug users and transfusion of blood and blood products.
- Sexual transmission is low.
- Complications include liver cirrhosis and hepatocellular carcinoma.
- Treatment is with interferon-α and ribavarin.

Hepatomegaly

Describe your clinical findings

On examination, there is a mass in the right upper quadrant. It moves with respiration and is dull to percussion. I cannot get above it. It is … cm below the right costal margin. This patient has hepatomegaly.

Comment on whether the liver is:

- Smooth or knobbly
- Pulsatile in tricuspid regurgitation

What are the causes of hepatomegaly?

- Cirrhosis – look for signs of chronic liver disease
- Carcinoma – usually secondary tumours, rarely primary tumours – the liver is often hard with a knobbly or nodular edge
- CCF – liver is firm, smooth and may be pulsatile if tricuspid regurgitation is present
- Infections – hepatitis A, B or C, EBV, leptospirosis, pyogenic or amoebic abscess
- Metabolic causes – haemochromatosis, Wilson's disease
- PBC
- Lymphoproliferative disorders
- Sarcoidosis
- Amyloidosis
- Budd–Chiari syndrome

How do you investigate hepatomegaly?

- See investigations for liver cirrhosis

When can the liver be palpable below the right costal margin without being enlarged?

- Emphysema
- Reidel's lobe
- Right-sided pleural effusion

What is Budd–Chiari syndrome?

- This is characterized by thrombosis of the hepatic veins resulting in:
  - abdominal pain
  - ascites
  - hepatomegaly
- Jaundice is usually absent.
- There are no cutaneous features of liver disease initially owing to the rapid onset of liver failure.
- The liver is smoothly enlarged and tender.

What are the causes of Budd–Chiari syndrome?

- Hypercoagulable states:
  - pregnancy
  - contraceptive pill
  - PRV
  - essential thrombocythaemia
  - antiphospholipid syndrome
  - protein C, protein S or antithrombin III deficiency
- Hepatocellular carcinoma
- Hepatic infections such as hydatid disease
- Renal and adrenal tumours
- Congenital venous webs

How do you investigate such patients?

- Liver biopsy
- USS of abdomen
- CT scan of abdomen

How would you manage such a patient?

- Surgery to correct congenital webs
- Anticoagulation
- Liver transplantation

Splenomegaly

Describe your clinical findings

On examination, this patient has a mass in the left upper quadrant of the abdomen. It is … cm below the left costal margin. I cannot get above the mass, and it is dull to percussion. It has a notch and does not ballot. It moves diagonally across the abdomen on inspiration.

This patient has splenomegaly. I would like to complete my examination by checking for lymphadenopathy in the axillae, cervical and inguinal areas.

What are the causes of splenomegaly?

Massive splenomegaly

- Myeloproliferative disorders – myelofibrosis, CML
- Malaria
- Kala-azar
- Gaucher's disease

Moderate and mild splenomegaly

- Portal hypertension due to liver cirrhosis
- Lymphoproliferative disorders – lymphoma and CLL

- Viral hepatitis
- Brucellosis
- Sarcoidosis
- ITP
- PRV
- Felty's syndrome
- Haemolytic anaemia (triad of jaundice, anaemia and splenomegaly)

How would you investigate this patient?

Blood tests

- FBC
- Blood film
- Viral serology

Imaging

- USS of abdomen

Other tests

- Lymph node biopsy
- Bone marrow aspirate and trephine

What are the indications for splenectomy?

- Ruptured spleen
- ITP not controlled by steroids
- Hereditary spherocytosis
- Symptoms due to massive organomegaly

What follow up do patients with splenectomy need?

- Vaccination against encapsulated bacteria:
  - pneumococcus
  - meningococcus
  - *H. influenzae*
- Prophylactic penicillin
- Medic alert bracelet

What is Felty's syndrome?

- This describes the association of rheumatoid arthritis with:
  - splenomegaly
  - neutropenia
  - lymphadenopathy

What are the lymphoproliferative disorders?

- ALL
- CLL
- Lymphoma

- Multiple myeloma
- Waldenstrom's macroglobulinaemia

What are the myeloproliferative disorders?

- AML
- CML
- Myelofibrosis
- PRV
- Essential thrombocytopaenia

What is the genetic abnormality found in CML?

- CML results from a reciprocal translocation between chromosomes 9 and 22 of the Philadelphia chromosome.
- The oncogene ABL is translocated from chromosome 9 to the BCR point on chromosome 22. ABL codes for a tyrosine kinase. This translocation results in aberrant tyrosine kinase activity, which leads to an acceleration in the growth and differentiation of the myeloid line.

How is CML diagnosed?

- Raised WCC
- Blood film shows large numbers of granulocytes and basophils
- Bone marrow is hypercellular with granulocytic hyperplasia
- Cytogenetic studies show Philadelphia chromosome

How is CML treated?

- Bone marrow transplant
- Tyrosine kinase inhibitors
- Autologous stem cell transplantation
- Interferon-α
- Hydroxyurea

Hepatosplenomegaly

Describe your clinical findings

On examination the liver is palpable … cm below the right costal margin and the spleen is enlarged at … cm below the left costal margin.

This patient has hepatosplenomegaly.

What are the causes of hepatosplenomegaly?

- Myeloproliferative disease
- Lymphoproliferative disease
- Cirrhosis with portal hypertension due to alcoholic liver disease or PBC
- Infectious causes:
  - hepatitis B or C
  - Epstein–Barr virus (EBV)
  - Cytomegalo virus (CMV)

- brucellosis
- leptospirosis
- toxoplasmosis
- malaria
- Infiltrative disorders:
  - amyloidosis
  - sarcoidosis
  - Gaucher's disease
  - glycogen storage disorders

Ascites

Describe your clinical findings

On examination there is generalized swelling of the abdomen. The umbilicus is everted. There is shifting dullness and a fluid thrill is present.

These findings suggest that the patient has abdominal ascites.

What are the other causes of a distended abdomen?

- Fat
- Fluid
- Faeces
- Flatus
- Fetus

What are the causes of ascites?

- Cirrhosis with portal hypertension
- Carcinoma
- Congestive cardiac failure (CCF)
- Hypoalbuminaemic states such as nephrotic syndrome
- TB
- Hypothyroidism
- Meigs' syndrome
- Constrictive pericarditis

How would you investigate this patient?

- Blood tests including liver screen
- USS of liver
- Ascitic tap
- Liver biopsy if needed

What tests would you perform on your sample of ascites?

- Cell count and differential
- Protein level
- Albumin level
- Amylase level
- Cytology
- Gram staining

What causes transudate and exudate ascites?

Transudate	Exudate
• Portal hypertension with cirrhosis	• Malignancy
• CCF	• TB
• Nephrotic syndrome	• Pancreatitis
• Hypothyroidism	
• Budd–Chiari syndrome	

What do you understand by the serum : ascites albumin gradient?

- Patients with normal portal pressures have a gradient < 1.1 g/dL.
- Patient with a gradient > 1.1 g/dL suggests portal hypertension. Transudate causes are likely.
- Patients with a gradient < 1.1 g/dL do not have portal hypertension, and exudate causes are likely.

How would you manage a patient with ascites?

- Identify and treat the underlying condition for liver disease.
- Restrict sodium intake.
- Restrict fluid intake if the sodium concentration falls to < 120mmol/L.
- Give diuretics such as furosemide and spironolactone.
- Provide therapeutic paracentesis to alleviate shortness of breath with infusion of salt-free albumin.

What treatment options would you consider in patients with recurrent or refractory ascites?

- TIPS (transjugular intrahepatic portosystemic shunt) – this creates an artificial channel in the liver that allows for communication between the portal vein (inflow) and the hepatic vein (outflow)
- Liver transplantation

What are the complications of ascites?

- Spontaneous bacterial peritonitis
- Shortness of breath due to the diaphragm being pushed up by large amounts of ascites

Primary biliary cirrhosis (PBC)

Describe your clinical findings

This lady appears to be jaundiced and has clubbing of her fingers. There is evidence of scratch marks on her arms. She has xanthelasma around the eyes and xanthomata around the joints. She has hepatomegaly with the liver measuring … cm below the right costal margin.

The most likely diagnosis is primary biliary cirrhosis.

What are the clinical features of PBC?

- Lethargy
- Steatorrhoea
- Pruritus and scratch marks
- Jaundice
- Clubbing
- Xanthomata
- Xanthelasma
- Hepatomegaly (± splenomegaly)
- Malabsorption of vitamin K (clotting abnormalities) and vitamin D (osteomalacia)

What do you know about PBC?

- Usually affects middle-aged women
- Autoimmune condition
- Associated with other conditions such as:
  - Sjögren's syndrome
  - systemic sclerosis
  - CREST syndrome (calcinosis, Raynaud's phenomenon, oesophageal dysmotility, sclerodactyly and telangiectasia)
  - RA
  - dermatomyosistis
  - Hashimoto's thyroiditis
  - coeliac disease
  - renal tubular acidosis
  - fibrosing alveolitis
  - SLE
  - myasthenia gravis
- Associated with an increased risk of hepatocellular cancer

How would you investigate this patient?

Bloods

- LFTs show raised ALP and GGT with normal ALT and AST
- Prolonged PT due to malabsorption of vitamin K caused by cholestasis
- Hypercholesterolaemia
- Antimitochondrial antibodies (especially the M2 subtype) are positive

Liver biopsy

- Shows increased copper deposition with fibrosis, cirrhosis and granulomas

Which drugs are used to control pruritus in these patients?

- Colestyramine
- Ursodeoxycholic acid

How do you manage patients with PBC?

Medical

- Corticosteroids
- Ciclosporin
- Azathioprine
- Methotrexate

Surgical

- Liver transplantation remains the only cure for PBC. Indications include:
  - intractable pruritus
  - bilirubin > 170µmol/L
  - intractable ascites
  - encephalopathy
  - spontaneous bacterial pruritus

What is PSC?

- Rare disease characterized by chronic inflammation and fibrosis of the bile duct
- Strong association with inflammatory bowel disease (particularly ulcerative colitis)
- Complications include chronic liver disease, infective cholangitis and cholangiocarcinoma
- Affects men more than women
- Liver transplant is often needed

What symptoms may patients experience?

- Pruritus
- Fatigue
- Fever
- Right upper quadrant pain

How would you investigate these patients?

Bloods

- Raised ALP and bilirubin
- Hypergammaglobulinaemia
- p-ANCA present in 50% of cases

ERCP

- Shows a 'beaded' appearance of the bile ducts

Haemochromatosis

Describe your clinical findings

This man has:

- Generalized hyperpigmentation
- Decreased body hair
- Gynaecomastia
- Stigmata of chronic liver disease (give examples) and
- Hepatomegaly ± splenomegaly

These findings suggest a diagnosis of haemochromatosis.

To complete my examination I would like to:

- Examine the cardiovascular system looking for cardiomyopathy and heart failure
- Examine for testicular atrophy
- Dipstick the urine looking for glucose

What do you know about haemochromatosis?

- Autosomal recessive condition with a carrier rate of 1 in 10 in Northern Europeans.
- Caused by mutations of the *HFE* gene on the short arm of chromosome 6.
- Results in increased iron absorption at the duodenum, and thus iron overload.
- Leads to iron deposits in major organs such as the skin, pancreas, liver, joints and anterior pituitary.
- Males may present at any age but females usually present after the menopause as iron loss in menstrual blood protects against iron overload and prevents the development of the disease.
- Homozygous individuals develop:
  - liver cirrhosis
  - hepatocellular carcinoma – patients with haemochromatosis are at 200-fold increased risk
  - diabetes (due to iron deposition in the pancreas and insulin resistance)
  - arthropathy affecting particularly the wrists, hips, knees and second and third MCPJs
  - cardiac disease including arrhythmias, cardiac failure and cardiomyopathy
  - hypogonadism due to iron deposition affecting hypothalamic–pituitary function.
- Asymptomatic relatives should undergo screening.

What is the prognosis?

- Reduced life expectancy if cirrhosis develops
- Normal life expectancy if cirrhosis is absent and the patient is compliant with treatment

What investigations would you do?

Bloods

- Transferrin saturation ↑
- Ferritin levels ↑

- TIBC↓
- FBG to screen for diabetes

Other tests

- Liver biopsy shows excessive iron storage
- Genetic testing
- ECG, CXR and echocardiography to evaluate cardiac failure

How to you manage patients with haemochromatosis?

- Patients should avoid alcohol.
- Patients should avoid uncooked shellfish as they are susceptible to septicaemia caused by the marine bacterium *Vibrio vulnificus*.
- Venesection of 500 mL weekly until haemoglobin is < 11 g/dL and serum ferritin < 10 μg/L (takes about 2 years) and then every 3 months thereafter prolongs life.

What other conditions are associated with generalized pigmentation?

- PBC
- Addison's disease
- Uraemia
- Malignancy

Wilson's disease

Describe your clinical findings

This patient has jaundice and hepatomegaly with the liver measuring … cm below the right costal margin. Examination of his eyes shows a Kayser–Fleischer ring. These features suggest a diagnosis of Wilson's disease.

What do you know about Wilson's disease?

- Autosomal recessive – defect on chromosome 13
- Often associated with a family history of consanguinity
- Results in excessive absorption of copper from the small intestine with decreased excretion of copper from the liver
- Results in increased copper deposition in the brain, cornea, liver and kidney
- Lifelong treatment with penicillamine or trientine is needed to prevent copper deposits

What are the clinical features of the disease?

- Liver cirrhosis
- Haemolytic anaemia
- Sunflower cataracts and Kayser–Fleischer rings in the cornea
- Neurological manifestations – Parkinsonism, ataxia, tremor and chorea – due to basal ganglia copper deposition appear in young adulthood
- Psychiatric problems such as depression, anxiety and psychosis
- Renal tubular acidosis

What do you know about Kayser–Fleischer rings?

- This is a golden-brown pigmentation at the corneal limbus.
- The ring is most marked at the superior and inferior poles of the cornea.
- They result from copper deposition in Descemet's membrane in the cornea.
- They are also found in PBC and autoimmune hepatitis.

How would you investigate such a patient?

- Serum caeruloplasmin (copper-carrying protein) would be reduced
- Serum copper concentration may be increased, reduced or normal
- Urinary copper excretion would be increased
- Liver biopsy showing copper overload

Abdominal mass

Epigastric mass

Describe your clinical findings

On examination, there appears to be a hard, non-tender mass measuring … cm by … cm in the epigastrium. It does not move with respiration. There is (or is not) associated hepatomegaly.

What is your differential diagnosis?

- Carcinoma of the stomach
- Carcinoma of the pancreas
- Lymphoma

What is Troisier's sign?

- Troisier's sign describes the enlargement of left supraclavicular lymph nodes, which is considered pathognomonic of abdominal carcinoma, particularly gastric carcinoma.
- Virchow's node (an enlarged left supraclavicular lymph node) is the node commonly palpated to elicit Troisier's sign.
- Gastric carcinoma metastasizes to the left supraclavicular lymph node as the lymphatic system for most of the body drains into the left subclavian vein.

What is Courvoisier's law?

- Courvoisier's law states that in the presence of a palpable gall bladder, painless jaundice is unlikely to be caused by gallstones.
- Gallstones form over a long period of time and cause a shrunken, fibrotic gall bladder that does not distend easily.
- The gall bladder is enlarged in pathological conditions that result in the obstruction of the biliary tree over a short time, such as pancreatic malignancy.

Mass in the right iliac fossa

Describe your clinical findings.

On examination, there appears to be a hard, non-tender mass measuring … cm by … cm in the right iliac fossa. It does not move with respiration.

Comment on whether hepatosplenomegaly is present.

What is your differential diagnosis?

- Crohn's disease
- Carcinoma of the caecum
- Lymphoma
- Transplanted kidney
- Ileocaecal tuberculosis
- Appendicular abscess
- Carcinoma of the ovary
- Ileal carcinoid

Mass in the left iliac fossa

Describe your clinical findings

On examination, there appears to be a hard, non-tender mass measuring … cm by … cm in the left iliac fossa. It does not move with respiration.

Comment on whether hepatosplenomegaly is present.

What is your differential diagnosis?

- Diverticular abscess
- Carcinoma of the colon
- Carcinoma of the ovary
- Faecal mass
- Transplanted kidney

Inflammatory bowel disease

Describe your clinical findings

On examination, this young, thin male patient has several surgical scars on his abdomen. He has a hard, non-tender mass measuring … cm by … cm in the right iliac fossa. It does not move with respiration. There is no associated hepatosplenomegaly.

This patient may have a diagnosis of inflammatory bowel disease.

What are the common causes of inflammatory bowel disease?

- Crohn's disease
- Ulcerative colitis

What are the macroscopic features of Crohn's disease?

- Involves all bowel layers
- Can affect any part of the gastrointestinal tract – from the mouth to the anus

- Most commonly affects the terminal ileum
- Skip lesions – discontinuous sites of gastrointestinal tract affected
- Cobblestone ulceration
- Lead-pipe thickening
- Strictures
- Rose-thorn ulcers

What are the microscopic features of Crohn's disease?

- Transluminal inflammation
- Non-caseating granulomas

What are the macroscopic features of ulcerative colitis?

- Affects the colon only
- Pseudopolyps
- Contact bleeding
- Haustral loss due to shortening and thickening of the bowel wall

What are the microscopic features of ulcerative colitis?

- Affects the mucosa and submucosa
- Crypt abscesses and ulcer formation

How would you investigate a patient with bloody diarrhoea?

- Stool microscopy and culture to exclude an infective cause of diarrhoea
- Blood tests to check for anaemia and inflammatory markers (CRP and erythrocyte sedimentation rate, ESR)
- Abdominal radiograph to exclude:
  - small bowel obstruction in Crohn's disease
  - toxic dilatation in ulcerative colitis
- Colonoscopy and biopsy for histological confirmation of diagnosis
- Bowel contrast studies to check for strictures and fistulae in Crohn's disease
- Abdominal CT scan if needed

How would you manage a patient with inflammatory bowel disease?

Medical management

- Nutritional support and elemental diet in Crohn's disease
- Steroids
- Immunosuppressant drugs such as aminosalicyclates, azathioprine, ciclosporin, methotrexate
- Infliximab (chimeric antibody to tumour necrosis factor)
- Metronizadole in Crohn's disease for treatment of fistulas, abscesses and bacterial overgrowth

Indications for surgery

- Crohn's disease:
  - intestinal obstruction
  - toxic dilatation of the colon

- failure to respond to medical therapy
  - fistula, perforation or abscess formation
- Ulcerative colitis – surgery can be curative:
  - symptomatic relief
  - perforation
  - toxic dilatation
  - refractory colitis
  - colonic carcinoma

What are the bowel complications in inflammatory bowel disease?

Crohn's disease	Ulcerative colitis
Malabsorption	Malnutrition
Anaemia	Anaemia
Abscess	Perforation
Fistula to bowel, bladder or vagina	Colonic cancer
Strictures	Toxic dilatation
Intestinal obstruction	
Intestinal perforation	

Name some extragastrointestinal manifestations of inflammatory bowel disease

Gastrointestinal

- Gallstones
- PSC

Musculoskeletal

- Arthritis
- Sacroilitis

Skin

- Erythema nodosum
- Pyoderma gangrenosum

Eyes

- Iritis
- Scleritis
- Episcleritis

Other

- Renal stones and strictures
- Amyloidosis

Nephrotic syndrome

Describe your clinical findings

This patient has periorbital oedema, oedematous ankles and ascites.

These findings may be due to nephrotic syndrome.

What are the causes of nephrotic syndrome?

Renal causes	Systemic causes
Minimal change disease	SLE
Focal and segmental GN	HSP
Membranous GN	Diabetes
Mesangiocapillary GN	Amyloidosis
Drugs such as NSAIDs, captopril and penicillamine	
Metals such as gold, mercury and cadmium	

What are the features of nephrotic syndrome?

- Proteinuria (> 3.5 g of protein per day)
- Hypoalbuminaemia
- Hyperlipidaemia
- Oedema:
  - periorbital oedema, worse in the mornings
  - pitting oedema of ankles and legs
  - ascites
  - pleural effusion

How would you investigate such a patient?

- 24-hour urinary protein or urine albumin/creatinine
- Urine microscopy
- Blood tests to check U&E, LFTs, albumin, lipid profile, glucose and autoimmune screen, hepatitis B and C screen
- Renal biopsy

How do you manage such patients?

- Dietary modification with low sodium and fluid restriction
- Penicillin may be given prophylactically to prevent pneumococcal infection
- Subcutaneous heparin for the prevention of venous thromboses in the bed bound
- Control blood pressure with ACE inhibitors
- Treat the underlying cause
- Immunosuppression:
  - steroids
  - ciclosporin
  - cyclophosphamide

What are the complications of nephrotic syndrome?

Thrombosis

- DVT, PE and renal vein thrombosis
- Due to a hypercoagulable state resulting from urinary loss of antithrombin
- Treat with oral anticoagulants

Infection

- Due to renal loss of immunoglobulins
- Infection with encapsulated bacteria such as *H. influenzae* and *S. pneumoniae* can occur

Acute renal failure

- Fluid accumulation in the tissues leads to hypovolaemia and so reduces blood flow to the kidneys.

Malnutrition

- Due to protein deficiency

Hypercholesterolaemia

- Results in an increased risk of ischaemic heart disease

Palpable kidneys

Describe your clinical findings

On examination, there is a well-defined mass measuring ... cm by ... cm in the right (± left) flank. It is bimanually ballotable and moves with respiration. I can get above the mass and the percussion note is resonant above it. This suggests that the mass is a single (or bilateral) enlarged kidney.

I would like to complete my examination by measuring the patient's blood pressure and checking his urine for protein and blood.

Causes of unilateral enlargement

- Simple cysts
- Polycystic kidney disease with only one kidney palpable
- Renal cell carcinoma
- Hydronephrosis
- Hypertrophy of a single functioning kidney

Causes of bilateral enlargement

- Polycystic kidney disease (hepatomegaly due to polycystic liver disease may occur)
- Bilateral renal cell carcinoma
- Bilateral hydronephrosis
- Amyloidosis

How would you investigate this patient?

- Blood tests to check renal function
- Urine microscopy
- Urine culture
- USS of abdomen
- Consider:
  - renal biopsy
  - IVU to exclude obstruction if needed
  - abdominal CT scan to exclude malignancy
  - genetic studies to diagnose adult polycystic kidney disease (ADPKD)

Polycystic kidney disease

Describe your clinical findings

On examination, this patient has an arteriovenous fistula with a thrill and bruit. There is also an abdominal scar. There is a well-defined mass measuring … cm by … cm in the right and left flank. Each mass is bimanually ballotable and moves with respiration. I can get above it and the percussion note above it is resonant. This suggests the presence of bilaterally enlarged kidneys. The arteriovenous fistula suggests that the patient is being treated with haemodialysis. The abdominal scar suggests previous peritoneal dialysis.

The most likely diagnosis is polycystic kidney disease. I would like to complete my examination by measuring the patient's blood pressure and checking his urine for protein and blood.

What do you know about polycystic kidney disease?

- This can be an autosomal dominantly or recessively inherited condition.
- The autosomal dominant form is more common.
- The incidence is 1 in 1000.
- It results in cystic degeneration of the kidneys leading to renal failure.
- End-stage renal disease will develop by 40–60 years of age.

What symptoms do patients usually present with?

- Hypertension
- Abdominal pain
- Haematuria
- Renal failure
- Recurrent urinary tract infection

What extrarenal manifestations do you know about?

Cysts	Non-cystic
Pancreas	Berry aneurysms with increased risk of subarachnoid haemorrhage
Liver	Colonic diverticula
Ovaries	Abdominal hernias
Nervous system	Mitral valve prolapse causing palpitations and atypical chest pain

How do you manage such patients?

- Genetic counselling and screening of family members
- Nephrectomy
- Dialysis
- Renal transplant

In what other conditions do renal cysts occur?

- Multiple simple cysts
- Tuberous sclerosis
- Von Hippel–Lindau disease

Renal transplantation

Describe your clinical findings

On examination, this patient has gum hypertrophy, suggesting immunosuppressant treatment with ciclosporin. There is a scar in the right iliac fossa. There is a palpable, round mass under the scar which is most likely to be a kidney. This patient has had a renal transplant and is likely to be on ciclosporin.

Other clinical signs

- Cushingoid appearance due to steroid treatment
- Parathyroidectomy scar to treat renal bone disease
- Hearing aid may suggest Alport's syndrome
- Nephrectomy scar
- Bilateral flank masses suggest polycystic kidney disease

What are the most common causes for a renal transplant?

- Diabetic nephropathy
- Hypertensive renal disease
- Glomerulonephritis
- Polycystic kidney disease

What drugs are used post transplant?

- Steroids
- Immunosuppressant drugs such as ciclosporin, azathioprine and mycophenolate mofetil

What complications follow after renal transplantation?

- Rejection of the transplanted kidney
- Infection with CMV or *Pneumocystis* spp.
- Side effects of immunosuppressive drugs, such as hypertension with ciclosporin
- Recurrence of original disease
- Increased risk of lymphoma and skin malignancy (SCC increased 100-fold and BCC increased 10-fold)
- Increased risk of cardiovascular risk factors leading to premature MI and stroke:
  - hypertension
  - hyperlipidaemia

I STATION 2 HISTORY TAKING SKILLS

Case 1

Information for the candidate

Please read this letter from the patient's GP and then take a history from the patient.

Referral letter

> *Please see this 55-year-old lady who presents with a 3-month history of worsening chest pains. Apart from osteoarthritis of the right knee she is otherwise fit and well. Her BP is 130/80 mmHg.*
> *Kind regards*
> *Dr Chester Payne*

Brief for the actor

You are a 55-year-old mother of three children and for the past 3 months have suffered from episodes of discomfort in the central chest. This feels like a burning sensation moving up the chest. The symptoms are worse at night and you are now using several pillows to relieve the discomfort. You have experienced burping and belching and occasional nausea and vomiting. If asked, you think the symptoms are often related to eating. The pain is not worse with movement, breathing in or exercising. Your weight is stable, and if asked about other symptoms you have none. The only other medical problem is arthritis of the knee, and you have been taking ibuprofen for this. You smoke 10 cigarettes a day and drink about 10 units of alcohol a week. You work as a dinner lady at a local school.

Data gathering

Personal details

- Full name, date of birth and occupation

History of presenting complaint

- Enquire about the pain:
  - location

- radiation (aortic dissection to back, angina to neck, jaw and arm, gastro-oesophageal from epigastric area radiating up chest wall)
- nature of pain (*burning* in gastro-oesophageal reflux, *crushing* in angina/MI, *pleuritic* in pulmonary embolus, pericarditis and pleurisy)
- triggers (cardiac pain is worse with exertion, reflux is worse when lying flat at night, muscular pain is worse with movement or twisting)
- relieving factors (pericarditis settles when leaning forwards, cardiac or muscular pain eases with rest)
- duration
- natural history of the pain – establish time course, clarify whether it is getting better, worse or unchanged, ask if it comes and goes
- medications used for pain such as NSAIDS, GTN spray, antacids

- Associated symptoms, e.g. nausea or vomiting, sweating, palpitations, breathlessness, cough (sputum, haemoptysis), belching, dizziness, fever
- Assess the impact of the pain on lifestyle, work and recreation
- Check for risk factors
  - cardiac: smoking, personal and family history of cardiovascular disease, hypertension, diabetes, hypercholesterolaemia
  - gastro-oesophageal: smoking, alcohol, NSAIDs, obesity, caffeine, stress, history of peptic ulcer disease
  - PE: smoking, immobility, recent surgery, recent long-haul travel, neoplastic disease, personal or family history of DVT or PE

Medical history

- Enquire about history of osteoarthritis
- Rule out other medical history including those mentioned in risk factors above

Drug history

- Enquire about medication taken for osteoarthritis e.g. NSAIDS, COX-2 inhibitors
- Any other prescribed or over-the-counter drugs
- Ask about any drug allergies

Family history

- Of cardiovascular, respiratory or other disease

Social history

- Recreational drug use
- Alcohol intake
- Smoking currently or ex-smoker
- Family details
- Housing
- Elicit the psychological impact of the symptoms
- Clarify how independent she is and if she can perform activities of daily living herself

Systems review

- Weight loss
- Loss of appetite
- Fevers or night sweats

Interpretation and use of information gathered

- Differential diagnosis:
  - reflux oesophagitis
  - stable or unstable angina
  - MI
  - pericarditis
  - aortic stenosis
  - recurrent PEs
  - muscular pain
  - other abdominal causes, e.g. biliary colic, pancreatitis
- Address alcohol/smoking/NSAID use
- Agree on a plan of action with the patient

Discussion related to the case

Please present this patient's history

This 55-year-old dinner lady presents with a 3-month history of central chest discomfort, which is worse on lying flat and relieved by sitting up. The pain is described as a burning sensation that moves up the chest wall. She sometimes requires four pillows at night to relieve the symptoms. There is associated belching and a few episodes of nausea and vomiting. The pain sometimes comes on soon after eating. The pain is not related to exertion and tends to improve during the daytime. I note that she has used ibuprofen for her osteoarthritis for the past 5 months. She smokes 10 cigarettes a day and drinks 10 units of alcohol a week. There are no systemic symptoms of weight loss, fevers or loss of appetite and the bowels are normal with no melaena.

This patient has symptoms of gastro-oesophageal reflex, probably exacerbated by her long-term use of ibuprofen and smoking.

What investigations would you arrange to confirm your diagnosis?

- Bloods (FBC, U&E, LFT, GGT, and bone profile)
- Consider ECG and CXR according to the history
- Endoscopy
- Consider 24-hour oesophageal pH monitoring

What are the complications of gastro-oesophageal reflux disease?

- Reflux oesophagitis
- Oesophageal stricture
- Barrett's oesophagus
- Adenocarcinoma (complication of Barrett's disease)

How would you manage this patient?

Lifestyle changes

- Stop ibuprofen and consider an alternative analgesic that is not an NSAID
- Stop smoking
- Decrease alcohol intake
- Weight loss if relevant
- Raise the head of the bed
- Small regular meals not too soon before sleeping and cut down on spicy foods

Medical

- Antacids e.g. Gaviscon®
- Proton pump inhibitor e.g. Lansoprazole 15mg o.d. or Omeprazole 20mg o.d.
- H_2 blocker e.g. Ranitidine 150mg b.d.

Case 2

Information for the candidate

You are one of the junior doctors. This patient has been referred to the gastroenterology outpatient department. Please read this letter from the patient's GP and then take a history from the patient.

Referral letter

I would be grateful for your opinion on this 30-year-old gentleman with a 2-month history of loose watery diarrhoea. He has lost a stone in weight. His medical history is otherwise unremarkable.
Regards
Dr Mel Hina

Brief for the actor

You are a 30-year-old man presenting with 2 months of watery stools. You are visiting the toilet between four and six times a day. If asked, the stools have not been blood stained and you have not noted pus. You have suffered occasional crampy pains in the lower abdomen which are relieved by opening your bowels. The symptoms began a week after a trip to Lahore in Pakistan. You took all necessary precautions (including malaria prophylaxis, vaccinations and drinking bottled water) and stayed in a five-star hotel. You are eating a lot less nowadays and have lost a stone in weight over the last few weeks. You work as a sales assistant and are facing the prospect of redundancy, which has been playing a lot on your mind. You have no significant past medical history, are on no regular medications and there is no relevant family history.

Data gathering

Personal details

- Full name, date of birth and occupation

History of presenting complaint

- Enquire about the diarrhoea:
  - duration
  - natural history – onset, how long symptoms have been present, any changes
  - frequency
  - consistency and colour – watery, steatorrhoea
  - presence of mucus, pus or blood
  - melaena
  - incontinence
- Associated symptoms such as weight loss, abdominal pain, vomiting, bloating, diarrhoea alternating with constipation, urinary symptoms, tenesmus, loss of appetite or jaundice
- Exacerbating factors such as wheat, barley and rye in coeliac disease
- Travel history
- Fever or night sweats

Medical history

- Irritable bowel syndrome
- Inflammatory bowel disease
- Infections
- Diabetes mellitus
- Thyroid disease
- HIV status
- Radiotherapy to bowel
- Anal fissures or fistulas

Drug history

- Laxative use
- Weight loss agents such as orlistat
- Antacids
- Antibiotics
- Drug allergies
- Enquire about malaria prophylaxis and vaccination during foreign travel

Family history

- Gastrointestinal disease
- Endocrine disease
- Gastrointestinal cancer

Social history

- Recreational drug use
- Alcohol use
- Smoker or ex-smoker
- Unwell contacts

- Occupational history (such as food factory worker)
- Home circumstances

Systems review

- To determine non-gastrointestinal causes such as diabetes mellitus or thyroid disease

Interpretation and use of information gathered

- Differential diagnosis:
    - gastrointestinal causes such as IBD, IBS, coeliac disease, chronic pancreatitis, diverticular disease, colorectal cancer
    - infective causes such as amoebiasis, giardiasis, hydatid disease, TB and HIV
    - endocrine disorders such as thyrotoxicosis, levothyroxine therapy, diabetic autonomic neuropathy
    - iatrogenic causes such as laxatives, antibiotics, radiation enteropathy
- Agree on a plan of action with the patient
- Any significant psychosocial issues, e.g. stress/anxiety at work

Discussion related to the case

Please present this patient's history

This 30-year-old man presents with a 2-month history of loose watery motions, which occur up to six times a day. There is no steatorrhoea. This began suddenly 1 week after a trip to Lahore in Pakistan. He stayed in a five-star hotel and took general precautions including bottled water. His vaccination history is up to date and malaria prophylaxis was taken. He has lost 1 stone in weight. He complains of associated crampy lower abdominal pains relieved by defecation, but no fever or night sweats. Systems review is otherwise unremarkable as are family history, past history and drug history. He has been under significant stress at work in the past few weeks and faces the possibility of being made redundant.

What do you think is the most likely diagnosis?

- Given the association with third world travel, the most likely cause is infective such as amoebic dysentery or giardiasis.
- IBD should also be ruled out (as should cancer; however, this is less likely given the age of the patient).

How would you investigate this patient?

Bloods

- FBC, ESR, U&E, LFTs, CRP, TFTs, bone profile, glucose, vitamin B_{12} levels (checking for signs of malabsorption) and coeliac screen

Stool culture

- For parasites, ova and cysts

Colonoscopy

- Rule out IBD and colonic cancer

Case 3

Information for the candidate

You are in the general medical outpatients department. Please read this letter from the patient's GP and then take a history from the patient.

Referral letter

I would be grateful for your opinion on this 55-year-old lady who complains of several painful nodular skin lesions on her shins over the past 4 weeks. Upon routine blood testing her corrected calcium is 2.8 mmol/L. All other blood tests are normal. I would be grateful for your expertise in managing her.
Best wishes
Dr Kal Seemeya

Brief for the actor

You are a 55-year-old woman, who, until a few months ago, has been fit and well all her life. You went to the GP a month ago complaining of painful rashes on the legs. You take Ibuprofen for this, which seems to be working. Your GP did some blood tests and you were told that you have a 'high calcium'. If asked about other health problems, you have visited your GP a number of times over the past few months with various complaints. These include stomach pains, eye infections, dry eyes, joint pains and feeling down. You have experienced no weight loss or night sweats. You have also suffered from increasing breathlessness and a cough and you are limited by how far you can walk. Six months ago you walked unlimited distances but this has gradually reduced to 50 metres before you are short of breath. You are a non-smoker and drink occasionally.

Data gathering

Personal details

- Full name, date of birth, occupation, ethnicity

History of presenting complaint

- Enquire about the skin lesion:
  - duration
  - natural history – time course, onset, changes
  - changes in lesion – size, presence in other sites such as arms
  - previous episodes
- Enquire about the pain and if painkillers, such as NSAIDs, have been used
- Enquire about symptoms of hypercalcaemia
  - mental health – history of depression
  - abdominal symptoms – abdominal pains, dyspepsia, constipation, pancreatitis
  - urinary symptoms – renal colic
  - bone pain
- Systemic symptoms – fever, night sweats, weight loss, malaise

Systems review

- Any long periods of immobility
- Respiratory symptoms (breathlessness, cough, haemoptysis)
- Hyperthyroidism symptoms
- Breast lumps suggestive of malignancy
- Eyes (red eyes, dry eyes)
- Musculoskeletal (joint pains, swollen joints)
- Travel history
- Dietary history of calcium-containing products such as a high milk intake

Medical history

- Depression
- Hyperparathyroidism
- Sarcoidosis
- TB
- Cancer
- Calcium deficiency (may have been overtreated)
- Obstetric and gynaecology history including smears and mammograms

Drug history

- Vitamin D analogues
- Lithium
- Thiazide diuretics
- Drug allergies

Family history

- Endocrine disorders
- Malignancy

Social history

- Enquire about any exposure to illnesses such as TB
- Smoking history
- Alcohol intake
- Family and living circumstances

Interpretation and use of information gathered

- Consider the causes of hypercalcaemia in general:
  - sarcoidosis
  - malignancy such as lymphoma, myeloma, bronchial, breast, bowel cancers
  - TB
  - hyperparathyroidism – primary and tertiary
  - ingestion – increased vitamin D intake, milk–alkali syndrome, drugs
  - prolonged immobility
  - endocrine – Addison's disease and hyperthyroidism

   - Paget's disease
   - familial hypocalciuric hypercalcaemia
- Consider which of these causes would also present with erythema nodosum:
   - sarcoidosis
   - TB (although less likely in this patient given the overall clinical picture)

For other causes of erythema nodosum, see Station 5, Case 2, p. 196.

Discussion related to the case

Please present this patient's history

This 55-year-old woman presents with a 6-week history of painful, nodular lesions affecting the shins. She has taken ibuprofen which has helped the pain and the skin lesions are now resolving. They are not located anywhere else and she has not had them in the past. Routine blood tests by her GP revealed hypercalcaemia. She has a recent history of abdominal pain and low mood. There is decreasing exercise tolerance due to breathlessness (unlimited 6 months ago, now 50 metres) and cough with no haemoptysis. Of note, she has been treated in the past year for conjunctivitis, complains of dry eyes and does suffer from occasional joint pains. There is no weight loss or night sweats. The remainder of the medical history and drug history are unremarkable. Mammograms and smears are up to date and negative. She is a non-smoker and drinks 5 units alcohol a week.

What do you think is the most likely diagnosis and why?

- Sarcoidosis, as suggested by the combination of erythema nodosum, worsening respiratory symptoms, eye signs, joint pains and hypercalcaemia

What investigations would you carry out in this patient?

Bloods

- FBC, ESR, U&E, LFTs, CRP, TFT, PTH and bone profile
- Serum ACE – more useful in monitoring response to therapy

Consider sputum cultures

- For Ziehl–Neelsen staining and TB culture

Other

- Consider the TB ELISPOT test

Chest radiograph

- Looking for hilar adenopathy, apical involvement or other signs of malignancy

Transbronchial biopsy

- Along with the CXR can provide a diagnosis of sarcoid in the majority of patients

Lung function testing

- For evidence of restrictive lung deficit due to fibrosis

Consider skin biopsy

- To confirm erythema nodosum

If this turns out to be sarcoidosis, what drugs may be useful in her management?

- Depending on the extent of involvement, prednisolone therapy may be commenced. Patients often have a good response.

Case 4

Information for the candidate

You are seeing patients in neurology outpatients. Your next patient has come to see you. Please read the GP letter and then take a history from this patient.

Referral letter

Please assess this 40-year-old gentleman who complains of new-onset intense headaches over the past 7 months. Blood pressure is 130/75 mmHg and examination of cranial nerves is unremarkable. He has tried various analgesics including ibuprofen and co-codamol with minimal effect.
Thanks for your input
Dr May Grane

Brief for the actor

You are a 40-year-old man who presented to your GP recently with episodes of severe headaches for the past 7 months. These seem to come out of the blue sometimes and can become so severe that it can wake you from sleep. The pain is located at the back of the left eye and moves to the cheek. The pain will come on and off for a few days, after which it may settle for a few weeks only to come back. The attacks last up to 40 minutes at a time. You have no other symptoms except that during the attacks the left eye becomes watery. Painkillers do not work. You have no other medical history and are a non-smoker and do not drink alcohol.

Data gathering

Personal details

- Full name, date of birth, occupation

History of presenting complaint

- Enquire about the headaches:
  - location
  - duration
  - natural history – time course, onset, ask if it comes and goes, e.g. in clusters
  - radiation – neck, band-like around the head (tension headache), facial involvement (trigeminal neuralgia, cluster headache)
  - nature – throbbing, sharp, intense
  - onset – sudden, 'vice-like' (subarachnoid haemorrhage), gradual onset
  - previous history of the headaches
- Enquire about analgesia taken – detailed enquiry about how often used, strengths, preparations

- Triggers, e.g. stress, tiredness, dietary factors
- Relieving factors, e.g. analgesia, rest
- Enquire about associations:
  - visual symptoms – blurring, loss of vision, zig-zags/lines in front of field, sensitivity to light (migraine)
  - nausea and vomiting
  - aura preceding the headaches (migraine)
  - altered consciousness, fits (epilepsy)
- Enquire about lifestyle factors and their relationship to the headaches, e.g. alcohol, caffeine, sleep and daily routine

Systems review

- Fever
- Weight loss
- Malaise
- Respiratory tract symptoms

Medical history

- Depression or anxiety
- Migraine
- Neurological disorders
- Hypertension
- Epilepsy
- Eyesight and recent eye test
- ENT-related problems, e.g. ears and teeth

Drug history

- Antidepressants
- Use of migraine medication, e.g. sumatriptan
- Consider analgesic overuse

Family history

- Brain tumours
- Migraine

Social history

- Recreational drug use
- Smoking and alcohol
- Detailed social history and effect of headaches on life at work, family and mood

Interpretation and use of information gathered

- Differential diagnosis:
  - migraine
  - tension headache

- cluster headache
- alcohol withdrawal headache
- benign intracranial hypertension
- sinusitis
- otitis media
- neoplastic, e.g. pituitary tumour
- temporal arteritis (less likely in a young person)
- cerebral thrombosis – venous or saggital sinus thrombosis
- subarachnoid or intracerebral haemorrhage
- meningitis (more likely acute presentations)

- Address psychosocial factors

Discussion related to the case

Please present this patient's history

This 40-year-old man presents with a 7-month history of bouts of severe left retro-orbital pain radiating to the cheek, sometimes waking him from sleep. The pain occurs on a daily basis for a few days at a time and tends to settle for up to a few weeks before recurring. The episodes usually last for 40 minutes. Ibuprofen and co-codamol are ineffective at terminating these attacks. There is an associated watering of the left eye during the attacks, but no visual symptoms, no nausea or vomiting and no aura. The patient is otherwise fit and well and apart from the analgesia is on no prescribed medication.

What do you think is the most likely diagnosis?

- Cluster headache

How would you manage this patient?

- Explain that this is unlikely to be anything serious and that analgesia is not usually effective in this condition
- Offer information in the form of leaflets to ensure better understanding
- Consider high-flow oxygen inhalation for acute cluster headache
- Prophylaxis with β-blockers, calcium channel blockers or lithium

Is there a specific investigation you would carry out in this patient?

- CT scanning to rule out a brain tumour
- Although the history is classic for cluster headache, one needs to be alert to the fact that these headaches are of relatively recent onset in a 40-year-old man

Case 5

Information for the candidate

You are one of the junior doctors in a respiratory outpatients clinic. Your consultant has asked you to see this next patient who has been referred in by his GP on a 2 week cancer wait.

Referral letter

> *Please assess this 67-year-old gentleman who complains of several episodes of haemoptysis over the past 3 months. He has a history of asthma and hypertension and is taking amlodipine 5 mg daily and salbutamol inhaler p.r.n. (when required). He is a lifelong smoker. Please see and advise.*
> *Dr Carl Synoma*

Brief for the actor

You are a 67-year-old retired salesman. You presented to your GP 2 weeks ago having had approximately five episodes of coughing up blood. If asked about the quantity of blood, there has been approximately a teaspoon's worth each time. You also noticed feeling generally unwell, with loss of appetite and people have commented that you have lost weight in the past 3 months. According to the scales, you think the weight loss could be about 1 stone. In the last 5 years you have suffered from increasing breathlessness and find it difficult to manage steep hills. Over this interval, the distance you can walk without feeling breathless has decreased to 50 metres. You have smoked 20 cigarettes a day since the age of 15 and have had no other medical problems prior to this, except admission for pneumonia on two occasions. If asked, you have not had any exposure to industrial chemicals. You are a retired salesman. You have not travelled abroad for over a decade and can answer 'no' to any other question about symptoms.

Data gathering

Personal details

- Full name, date of birth, occupation and ethnicity

History of presenting complaint

- Enquire about haemoptysis:
  - duration
  - frequency of episodes
  - quantity of blood loss – specks, teaspoonful, egg cupful, etc.
  - colour of blood – bright red, frank blood, frothy pink – ask if there is sputum and if the blood is separate or mixed in with or without clots
  - sputum production – if so enquire about consistency and colour
  - previous history of haemoptysis
- Enquire about associations:
  - cough – ask about history of cough, sputum, fever, nocturnal
  - breathlessness – ask about exercise tolerance, orthopnoea, PND (heart failure)
  - wheeze (COPD/asthma or cardiac asthma)
  - chest pain – enquire about cardiac chest pain and pleuritic pain (PE)
  - other cardiac symptoms – ankle swelling, syncope
  - upper airway symptoms including nosebleeds (Wegner's granulomatosis)
  - calf pain or swelling (DVT)
- Enquire about PE risk factors:
  - smoking (take detailed history, including pack-years)

- recent surgery
- immobility
- obesity
- history of PE or DVT

Systemic review

- Fever
- Night sweats
- Weight loss
- Malaise

Travel history and previous residence

- Third world travel
- Take detailed travel history
- Enquire about other countries lived in the past
- Enquire about contacts visiting from other countries, especially from third world countries, and unwell contacts including infection with TB

Medical history

- TB
- Malignancy
- Recurrent chest infections
- COPD
- PE
- Clotting disorders
- Other causes of immunocompromise including HIV risk factors

Drug history

- Anticoagulants
- NSAIDs

Family history

- TB
- Malignancy especially bronchial carcinoma

Social history

- Housing conditions
- Alcohol intake
- Smoking in pack-years
- Detailed social history including occupational history and occupational exposures, e.g. asbestos

Interpretation and use of information gathered

- Differential diagnosis:
  - bronchial carcinoma
  - TB
  - bronchiectasis

  - pneumonia
  - PE
  - pulmonary oedema
  - Wegner's granulomatosis
  - arteriovenous malformations
  - clotting disorders
  - anticoagulants
- Answer the patient's enquiries about likely diagnosis and investigations

Discussion related to the case

Please present this patient's history

- This 67-year-old man, who has smoked 20 cigarettes a day for the past 52 years, presents with a 3-month history of haemoptysis. He has experienced at least five such episodes, each comprising approximately a teaspoon of fresh red blood. He also complains of weight loss of 1 stone along with loss of appetite. The patient has for the past 5 years had a constant cough productive of yellow sputum, and I note two admissions in that time for pneumonia. There has been gradual reduction in exercise tolerance over the past 5 years to 50 metres and he also has difficulty managing sharp inclines. There is no chest pain and no other cardiac or respiratory symptoms of note and no other PE risk factors. The patient has had no recent third world travel and no exposure to TB. The patient is a retired salesman and had no exposure to asbestos.

What are the most likely diagnoses?

- Bronchial carcinoma
- Bronchiectasis
- COPD exacerbation*

*According to the detailed history that you will have taken, this patient seems to have COPD and not asthma (as is written in the referral letter). This case highlights the importance of not assuming that everything in the referral letter is correct and of taking a detailed history.

What investigations would you perform in this patient?

Bloods

- U&E, FBC, LFTs, bone profile and clotting

Sputum

- Microscopy, culture and sensitivity
- Ziehl–Neelsen staining
- Sputum cytology

Chest radiograph

- Pulmonary oedema, signs of TB, malignancy, infection

Bronchoscopy

- The examiners may focus on this in some detail, asking you to explain the reason for the procedure to the patient, as well as how it is performed, the risks and complications.

Other

- TB ELISPOT test

CT scan of thorax

- To exclude malignancy, TB and PE

Case 6

Information for the candidate

You are in neurology outpatients. Your next patient has come to see you. Please read the letter from the GP and then take a history from this patient.

Referral letter

Please assess this 50-year-old gentleman who presents with two tonic–clonic seizures within the past 4 weeks, each lasting up to 5 minutes. Of note, he has a history of depression and drinks 50–60 units of alcohol a week. He takes amitriptyline 25 mg at night. Neurological examination is normal. I am worried there could be a sinister cause for these fits.
Dr Frank Petit

Brief for the actor

You are a 50-year-old man who has presented with two fits within the past month. You lost consciousness when these occurred and eventually woke to hear your daughter calling out for you. You felt confused and disorientated for over an hour after each fit with muscle aches and fatigue. Your daughter explained that you made 'jerky movements' of the arms and legs during the fit and your eyes rolled back. You drink on average seven pints a night but have a binge of a further five whisky shots on Friday and Saturday evening. If asked, you do not recall having had a head injury or fall. The fits occurred after particularly 'heavy nights on the alcohol'. You have a past medical history of depression and have been taking antidepressants for the past 5 years. Your wife died of breast cancer 6 years ago, and soon after that you started feeling down. Your mood has been generally stable on the antidepressants.

Data gathering

Personal details

- Full name, date of birth and occupation

History of presenting complaint

- Enquire about the seizures:
  - confirm that they were seizures
  - presence of witnesses
  - circumstances at the time, location
  - ask if the patient lost consciousness and, if so, for how long
  - type of seizure, e.g. tonic–clonic, myoclonic, absence

    - duration
    - previous history of seizures
    - ask about tongue biting, faecal and urinary incontinence
    - post-ictal symptoms such as headache, confusion, drowsiness
    - triggers such as stress, drugs, alcohol, bright lights
    - termination of seizures – ask if spontaneous or if drugs were administered
- Enquire about associations:
    - headaches
    - visual symptoms
    - nausea and vomiting
    - aura preceding the seizures, e.g. déjà vu
    - palpitations
    - recent falls or head injuries
- Enquire about lifestyle factors:
    - alcohol history – include enquiry about withdrawal symptoms and eye openers
    - sleep and daily routine
    - recreational drug use, e.g. amphetamines, opiate-based drugs

Systemic review

- Fever
- Weight loss
- Malaise

Past medical history

- Epilepsy
- Cardiac arrhythmias
- Liver disease
- Depression – enquire about this in detail. Ask if there was any overdose taken and what treatments are taken for the depression

Drug history

- Tricyclic and other antidepressants
- Lithium
- Neuroleptics
- Oral hypoglycaemics and insulin use

Family history

- Neurological disorders
- Brain tumours

Social history

- Living circumstances
- Family and housing circumstances

- Alcohol intake and how it affects him on a daily basis. Perform the CAGE questionnaire if appropriate. An answer of 'yes' to two or more of the following questions is clinically significant for a drinking problem:
  - Do you ever feel you should **cut** down your drinking?
  - Do you get **annoyed** if people complain about your drinking?
  - Do you ever feel **guilty** about your drinking?
  - Do you ever have an **eye opener** in the morning?
- Smoking history
- Occupational history
- Forensic history

Interpretation and use of information gathered

- Differential diagnosis of seizures:
  - alcohol withdrawal fits
  - seizures due to tricyclic use
  - primary epilepsy
  - meningoencephalitis
  - neoplastic from primary brain tumour or metastases
  - subarachnoid haemorrhage
  - metabolic due to electrolyte imbalance, hypoglycaemia (from Addison's disease, liver failure or insulinoma) or hypoxia
  - drugs such as amphetamines or narcotics

Discussion related to the case

Please present this patient's history

This 50-year-old man presents with two new-onset seizures within the past month. These were both witnessed by his daughter. The description is that of a tonic–clonic seizure, each lasting about 5 minutes and settling spontaneously. Post-ictally, the patient was confused with symptoms of fatigue and muscle aches. The main association is that the patent had a binge on alcohol the night before the two seizures. He cannot recall a head injury. The patient drinks 60 units of alcohol per week, has several binges and does describe symptoms of tremor and irritability when he has long periods of abstinence. The patient has been treated for depression for the past 5 years and takes amitriptyline 25 mg at night. He denies any recreational drug use and has never overdosed on medication.

Discuss the likely factors in this patient's seizures

According to the history, this patient's seizures are likely to have a multifactorial basis, which needs exploring. The main factors are as follows:

- Heavy alcohol intake: the seizures followed particularly heavy binges, which would suggest a withdrawal seizure.
- Use of tricyclic antidepressants: these lower the threshold for seizures. Of note in this patient, he has remained on the same dose of amitriptyline for 5 years, which makes this a less likely option. Obviously one needs to be open to the possibility of overdose, although the patient denies this.

- The possibility of liver disease needs to be considered: hepatic encephalopathy is more likely to present acutely and the patient would have stigmata of liver disease.

What investigations would you perform in this patient?

Bloods
- U&E, FBC, LFTs, GGT, ESR, CRP, calcium, albumin, glucose and clotting

CXR
- For signs of infection and malignancy

ECG
- Helps distinguish epilepsy from other causes of blackout spells

CT scan or MRI of the brain
- To rule out brain tumour/subdural haematoma
- MRI would identify aneurysm and tumour

How would you manage this patient?

- Arrange the above investigations urgently and follow up.
- Address heavy alcohol intake:
  - explain the complications of heavy alcohol intake
  - offer referral for alcohol support and detoxification therapy
  - thiamine and multivitamin supplements
- Consider weaning off amitriptyline and replacing with a more appropriate antidepressant.
- Explain to the examiner that you would take advice from a psychiatrist about this.

Note This case is an example of a condition in which the main symptom could have several causes. It is important to take a detailed history, as for any station, and devise a list of problems, which shows the examiner that you have considered all the possibilities.

Case 7

Information for the candidate

You are the doctor in endocrine outpatients. The next patient has type II diabetes and has been referred in by the GP. Please read the GP's letter and then take a history from this patient.

Referral letter

Please could you assess this 45-year-old gentleman who was diagnosed with type II diabetes 6 months ago. I started treatment with metformin and have titrated that up to 850 mg t.d.s. The patient is also on gliclazide 160 mg b.d. Unfortunately his HbA_{1c} has only come down from 11 to 9. The patient has a BMI [body mass index] of 33 and his BP [blood pressure] is 150/95 mmHg. The last cholesterol level was 5.5 mmol/L.
I would be most grateful for your input
Dr B.M. Stix

Brief for the actor

You are a 45-year-old man. Your GP has referred you to the outpatients clinic because your diabetes is not well controlled. You were diagnosed with diabetes 6 months ago. You work in a warehouse and do frequent night shifts, which can be very tiring. Due to your hectic lifestye and erratic hours, you sometimes forget to take your medication. You have been told to lose weight and stop smoking and drinking, but you do not see why this is important and are not familiar with the consequences of being diabetic. You have missed diabetic checks at your GP surgery and not attended annual eye checks. You find that these habits provide you with pleasure in view of your hectic lifestyle. You smoke 10 cigarettes a day and drink 15 units of alcohol a week. You are married and have two teenage children at school. Your father passed away from a heart attack aged 55.

Data gathering

Personal details

- Full name, date of birth and occupation

History of presenting complaint

- Enquire about type II diabetes:
  - initial presentation to GP
  - clarify the non-pharmacological measures the patient has taken (if any)
  - enquire as to input from other health professionals such as the dietitian or podiatrist
- Enquire about complications:
  - microvascular – feet, kidneys, eyes
  - macrovascular – cardiac, brain, peripheral vascular disease
  - symptoms of neuropathy, e.g. burning feet, loss of sensation
- Ask about routine checks:
  - retinopathy screening
  - urine microalbumin checks
  - foot checks
  - blood pressure checks
- Ask about self-monitoring of blood sugars
- Enquire about lifestyle issues and the impact of diabetes on lifestyle:
  - diet – sugars, saturated fats, fried foods
  - alcohol history
  - smoking history
  - exercise and weight reduction
- Ask about other cardiovascular risk factors:
  - hypercholesterolaemia
  - past history of heart disease, stroke or peripheral vascular disease
  - family history of cardiovascular diseases
- Check patient understanding:
  - reason for referral, explanation of HAB1c

- complications – importance of stopping smoking/alcohol, significance of weight reduction
- opportunity to ask questions

Medical history

- Complications of diabetes
- Consider secondary causes of diabetes, e.g. pancreatitis

Drug history

- Clarify compliance with medication
- Adverse reactions
- Any other problems with taking medication, e.g. forgetting to take, inconvenience of taking at work
- Oral hypoglycaemics such as metformin and gliclazide
- Antihypertensives
- Statins
- Aspirin
- Possible use of diabetogenic drugs, e.g. steroids, β-blockers, thiazides

Family history

- Type II diabetes
- Cardiovascular disease

Social history

- Alcohol intake and smoking history
- Daily routine
- Occupational history

Interpretation and use of information gathered

- Formulate a list of problems for the patient.
- Consider the effectiveness of current treatments and what scope there is to optimize oral diabetic control.
- Discuss the possibility of insulin or other injectable agents.
- Consider cardiac risk factor control and lifestyle modification.
- Address compliance issues and patient understanding.

Discussion related to the case

Please present this patient's history

This 45-year-old man was diagnosed with type II diabetes on routine blood testing 6 months ago. He now takes metformin and gliclazide. Unfortunately there has been little improvement in HbA_{1c} readings (11 to 9). Mr Stix works shifts at a warehouse and admits to not always taking medication when on night shifts. He was not fully aware of the complications of diabetes, and I have explained these to him. He has not had formal eye testing nor urine microalbumin checks. His risk factors for cardiovascular disease are as follows: smoker 10 cigarettes a day, hypertension, cholesterol 5.5 mmol/L, high BMI and family history of heart disease (father died of MI, aged 55). He drinks 15 units of alcohol per week. He is adamant that he will not try insulin.

In summary, this patient has poorly controlled type II diabetes and several cardiac risk factors, and is currently on gliclazide and metformin.

What investigations would you carry out in this patient?

- Refer for retinal screening
- Urine microalbumin
- Routine ECG (in view of multiple risk factors)

What other drug treatments would you consider starting in this patient?

- The patient might benefit from a gliptin, e.g. sitagliptin, to improve HbA_{1c} control.
- Titrating up the ACE inhibitor would optimize the blood pressure as well slowing the progression of nephropathy. The National Institute for Health and Clinical Excellence (NICE) guidelines suggest keeping BP < 140/80 mmHg if there are no complications (otherwise < 130/80 mmHg).
- Statin therapy (aim for cholesterol < 4 mmol/L).
- Consider weight reduction treatment with orlistat.
- Discuss the prospect of insulin therapy if adequate control is not achieved.

What do you know about new agents used for the treatment of type II diabetes?

- Dipeptidyl peptidase 4 (DPP-4) inhibitors (sitagliptin, vildagliptin) prolong the activity of glucagon-like peptide 1 (GLP-1) – oral, not associated with weight loss or hypoglycaemia, used in second-line dual therapy.
- GLP-1 mimetics (exenatide, liraglutide) are associated with weight loss but not with hypoglycaemia – injection twice daily, used in third-line therapy.
- Thiazolidinediones (pioglitazone, rosiglitazone) – authorization was suspended in 2010 due to increased risk of heart attack and cerebrovascular accident (CVA).
- Long-acting insulin analogues (detemir, glargine) – injection.
- GLP-1 is secreted by ileal cells in response to carbohydrates, protein and lipids. It increases insulin secretion, suppresses glucagon secretion, slows gastric emptying and increases satiety. It is derived from proglucagon, hence its name, even though its actions are opposite to those of glucagon. It is rapidly metabolized (half-life 2 minutes) by DPP-4.

Table 5 Newer Diabetic Agents

Drug	Indications	Mode of action	Side effects	Route
Dipeptidyl peptidase 4 (DPP-4) inhibitors e.g. sitagliptin, vildagliptin	Second dual therapy (if metformin/ sulfonylurea not suitable) Sometimes triple therapy when insulin not suitable	Inhibit DPP-4, which increases insulin secretion and reduces glucagon secretion	No weight loss and no hypoglycaemia	Oral
GLP-1 mimetics e.g. exenatide, liraglutide	Used in third-line therapy with metformin and sulfonylurea	Increases insulin secretion, reduces glucagon secretion and slows gastric emptying	Weight loss but no hypoglycaemia	Subcutaneous injection
Long-acting insulin analogues e.g. detemir, glargine	Useful in those with tendency to hypoglycaemia	Structure is modified to delay absorption or prolong action	Hypoglycaemia	Subcutaneous injection
Thiazolidinediones e.g. pioglitazone	Same as DPP-4 inhibitors OR Addition to insulin therapy	Reduces peripheral insulin resistance leading to reduced blood glucose	Rosiglitazone has been withdrawn from the UK due to increased cardiovascular risk. MHRA safety alert concerning pioglitazone and risk of bladder cancer. There have also been saftey alerts regarding pioglitazone and cardiovascular safety. Liver impairment. Hypoglycaemia when used with sulfonlyurea.	Oral

Rationale for therapy

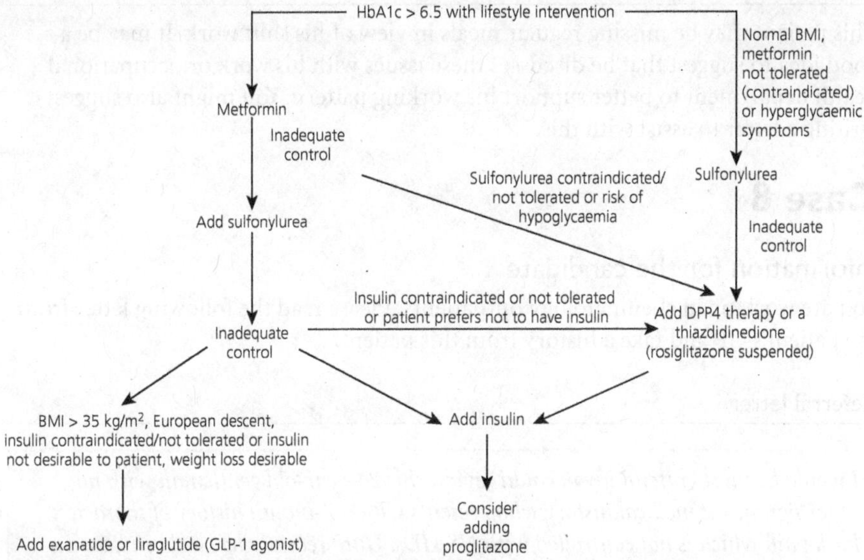

- Add insulin if inadequate control with above regimen.
- Stop DPP-4 inhibitor if HbA1c does not fall by 0.5% within 6 months.
- Stop the GLP-1 mimetic if HbA1c does not fall by 1% and there is < 3% weight loss within 6 months.
- Rosiglitazone was suspended by the European Medicines Agency in September 2010 because its benefits were no longer found to outweigh its risks.
- Although proglitazone is still available, a safety warning was issued in September 2011 by the Medicines and Healthcare Products Agency. It highlights the risk of bladder cancer with use of proglitazone.
- Proglitazone should only be continued if the HbA1c decreases by at least 0.5% within 6 months of initiating treatment.
- Further NICE guidance has been released stating that GLP-1 agonists can be used as dual therapy with metformin or sulfonylurea under certain circumstances. GLP-1 agonists may also be used as triple therapy alongside metformin and pioglitazone in certain situations.

Figure 2 **Rationale for therapy of diabetes. Based on National Institute for Health and Clinical Excellence. *Type 2 diabetes: newer agents for blood glucose control in type 2 diabetes*, NICE guideline CG66. London: NICE, 2008.**

What other management options would you pursue?

- There are multiple factors that need addressing in this patient, which could improve the patient's long-term outcome. I would adopt a multidisciplinary approach:
    - aggressive cardiac risk factor management
    - smoking cessation
    - alcohol reduction
    - dietitian
    - diabetic nurse input
    - diabetic retinopathy screen
    - weight reduction measures – exercise on prescription, goal setting to decrease BMI
    - podiatry input
    - support groups and follow-up

What social factors might be affecting this patient's diabetic control and what might you suggest?

This patient may be missing regular meals in view of his shift work. It may be a good idea to suggest that he discusses these issues with his work or occupational health department to better support his working pattern. You might also suggest writing a letter to assist with this.

Case 8

Information for the candidate

You are working in rheumatology outpatients. Please read the following letter from the patient's GP and take a history from this patient.

Referral letter

I would be most grateful if you could review this 24-year-old gentleman with no other significant medical history who presents with a 7-month history of thoracic back pain which is not controlled with NSAIDs. Until recently he has been keen on sports but has had to give them up due to the pain. Please review in your outpatients.
Kind regards
Dr Sye Atica

Brief for the actor

You are a 24-year-old man who went to his GP a month ago complaining of ongoing back pain. You have tried ibuprofen and diclofenac regularly with little effect. The pain is waking you up at night, and in the mornings your back can be quite stiff for up to 30 minutes. The pain is now present all the time. You notice that movement and activity makes the pain better and resting brings it on. You have also noticed niggles of pains in the right hip but are otherwise fit and well. You have had no fevers, night sweats or weight loss. You work in an office as a desk clerk and the pain is starting to affect you.

Data gathering

Personal details

- Full name, date of birth, occupation, ethnicity

History of presenting complaint

- Enquire about back pain:
  - location
  - duration
  - radiation, e.g. down the legs, to the anterior chest wall
  - nature of the pain
  - frequency of episodes
  - natural history of back pain over the last 7 months
  - night pain

  - ask about inflammatory symptoms, such as improvement with walking and movement, worse when resting, morning stiffness, fever
  - ask about mechanical symptoms, such as worse with movement, exercise, bending, sneezing, coughing and better with resting
  - explore any other triggers or exacerbating factors
  - history of analgesic use
  - treatments undertaken such as physiotherapy
- Ask about associated symptoms:
  - urinary retention, incomplete bladder emptying, faecal incontinence and saddle anaesthesia
  - joint pains affecting hips, knees, ankle, small joints of the hands and feet
  - gastrointestinal symptoms
  - genitourinary symptoms including testicular lumps
  - skin and eye signs
- Enquire about general lifestyle:
  - comparison of premorbid activity to now
  - explore the impact the back pain is having on his life
  - occupational history especially manual work

Travel history

- Third world travel
- Contact with TB

Medical history

- Previous back problems
- Ankylosing spondylitis
- TB
- Psoriasis
- Connective tissue disease

Drug history

- NSAIDs
- Steroid use

Family history

- TB
- Malignancy
- Ankylosing spondylitis

Social history

- Smoking and alcohol intake
- Occupational history
- Effect of back pain on daily activities
- Housing situation (house versus bungalow or flat, presence of stairs)

Systems review

- Fever
- Night sweats
- Weight loss
- Malaise
- Respiratory symptoms (cough and haemoptysis)

Interpretation and use of information gathered

- Differential diagnosis:
  - ankylosing spondylitis and seronegative arthritis
  - infective causes e.g. TB, abscess, infective discitis
  - malignancy, e.g. from a testicular tumour
  - prolapsed disc
  - fracture
  - spondylolisthesis
- Answer the patient's enquiries about likely diagnosis and investigations

Discussion related to the case

Please present this patient's history

This 24-year-old man presents with a 7-month history of worsening thoracic back pain which is now almost continuous. The patient has morning stiffness and night pain, which often wakes him from sleep. He has tried NSAIDs, which are becoming less effective. The pain is exacerbated by resting and relieved by movement. There has been no trauma. He has no constitutional symptoms, although he does describe an occasional ache in his right hip. He is previously fit and well and there is no significant medical history of note.

What do you think is the most likely diagnosis?

The patient has inflammatory back pain. At this age one would have to consider ankylosing spondylitis as the most likely diagnosis, although infective causes and malignancy need excluding.

What investigations would you carry out in this patient?

Bloods

- ESR, CRP, U&E, LFTs and bone profile
- RF and ANA

Thoracic and sacroiliac radiographs (anterior–posterior and lateral)

- These may be normal.
- Ankylosing spondylitis may have erosions/fuzziness in the sacroiliac joints in the early stages and periarticular sclerosis and flattening of vertebral bodies/fusion later on.

MRI

- Not usually indicated unless diagnostic uncertainty

What are the main treatments for ankylosing spondylitis?

- NSAIDs – this patient is likely to require indometacin
- Intensive physiotherapy and encouragement to remain active even during a flare-up

Case 9

Information for the candidate

You are the FY2 doctor in medical outpatients. You have been asked to see this next patient. Please read the GP's letter and then take a history from the patient.

Referral letter

Please could you review this 74-year-old gentleman in your outpatient clinic who has presented with two episodes of haematuria in the past 2 weeks. There is no other significant medical history and the patient is on no medications.
Kind regards
Dr Frank Heemat

Brief for the actor

You are a 74-year old man, who has experienced two recent episodes of fresh bright blood mixed in the urine. You have been fit and well all your life. If asked, you have noticed that your urine stream is slow and that there is dribbling after you empty your bladder. You also noted some occasional pain in the loins, but the episodes of blood in the urine were not accompanied by pain. You have no other symptoms. You worked as a civil servant until 65 and had no exposure to industrial chemicals.

Data gathering

Personal details

- Full name, date of birth and occupation

History of presenting complaint

- Enquire about haematuria:
  - confirm blood loss in the urine
  - quantity of blood in terms of pale pink urine or frank blood loss with clots
  - ask if there is frank blood loss mixed in with the stream, at the start of the stream, end of the stream or separate from the stream
  - confirm painless haematuria
  - ask if there have been any previous episodes
  - ask about any ingestions that may mimic haematuria such as rifampicin or beetroot

- Ask about associated symptoms:
  - urinary symptoms such as dysuria, frequency, nocturia, poor stream, post-terminal dribbling, loin pain, renal colic
  - abdominal symptoms
  - recent sore throat or upper respiratory tract infection
- Enquire about risk factors for bladder cancer:
  - smoking
  - occupational hazards such as working in the aniline dye or rubber industry
  - history of schistosomiasis infection
  - personal or family history of bladder cancer

Systemic review

- Fever
- Rigors
- Weight loss

Medical history

- Previous episodes of haematuria
- Renal disease
- Prostatic disease
- TB
- Hypertension

Drug history

- Anticoagulants
- Rifampicin

Family history

- Malignancy
- Polycystic kidney disease

Social history

- Occupation
- Travel abroad (including a history of bathing in lakes/rivers in Africa, the Middle East, India, South East Asia)
- Living circumstances
- Alcohol and smoking history

Interpretation and use of information gathered

- Differential diagnosis
  - malignancy of bladder, prostate or kidneys
  - infections such as schistosomiasis (*Schistosoma haematobium*) and TB
  - calculi
  - sickle cell disease

  - renal disease such as polycystic kidney disease, nephritic syndrome, papillary necrosis and IgA nephropathy
  - coagulation disorders
  - drugs, e.g. warfarin
  - trauma
  - intense exercise
- Consider false-positives:
  - haemoglobinuria
  - myoglobinuria
  - porphyria
- Answer the patient's enquiries about likely diagnosis and investigations
- Include an explanation of cystoscopy including its complications

Discussion related to the case

Please present this patient's history

This 74-year-old man presents with two episodes of painless haematuria. The blood was mixed into the urine and was bright red. The patient describes recent-onset intermittent loin pain with no radiation, which comes and goes, but there are no other urinary symptoms except for some hesitancy and post-terminal dribbling which he has experienced for over 5 years. There are no constitutional symptoms, including no night sweats and no weight loss. There is no other significant medical history, the patient is on no medication and has had no recent travel. He is a retired civil servant and has had no exposure to any industrial chemicals such as aniline dyes.

What condition would you want to rule out the most?

In a patient of this age with painless haematuria malignancy needs to be ruled out, particularly within the renal tract (bladder, prostate and renal canal in particular).

What investigations would you carry out in this patient?

Bloods

- U&E, FBC, LFTs, PSA, clotting screen and bone profile
- IgA levels

Urine

- MSU
- Urine cytology
- Urine microscopy, red cells and casts

Radiology

- Kidney–ureter–bladder radiograph
- USS of renal tract
- IVU
- CT scan of abdomen

Invasive tests

- Cystoscopy and biopsy, given the age of the patient, to exclude bladder cancer

Case 10

Information for the candidate

You are the medical doctor working on an acute medical take. Your next patient is a 25-year-old gentleman, Mr Jonathan Maynard, presenting with fever, muscle and joint aches. The triage nurse recorded the following observations:

Temperature 38.7 °C
BP = 122/76 mmHg
Pulse 102/minute
RR = 15/minute
Urine dipstick = negative.

Please take a history from this patient.

Brief for the actor

You are a 25-year old man, Jonathan Maynard, who has been unwell for the past 4 days. You have had high fevers, up to 39.5°C, along with symptoms of tiredness, mild headache, muscle and joint pains. You think you have a bad cold because you also have a slight runny nose. You started feeling unwell a week ago with general tiredness and have developed a fever over the last few days. You have no other significant medical history and take only cetirizine for hay fever. You are a non-smoker and drink alcohol socially. You work as a car salesman.

You only reveal the following information if specifically asked. You returned 3 days ago from a 2-month trip to Indonesia. You completed all your travel vaccinations prior to travelling but you decided against taking malaria prophylaxis because you hate taking tablets. You were not very good at using mosquito repellents and had a lot of bites over most of your body. You want the doctor to confirm that this is a virus and give you some pills and maybe a sick note for work. You are not expecting to be suffering from anything serious.

Data gathering

Personal details

- Full name, date of birth, occupation

History of presenting complaint

- Enquire about the fevers:
  - onset
  - duration
  - readings from a thermometer and any fluctuation e.g. spiking fevers
  - response to anti-pyretics
- Enquire about associated symptoms:
  - Systemic symptoms e.g. malaise, myalgia and arthralgia
  - Upper and lower respiratory tract symptoms
  - Abdominal symptoms i.e. pain, diarrhea, vomiting
  - Headache, rash, neck stiffness and photophobia
  - Urinary symptoms

- Travel history. Enquire specifically about any recent foreign travel, in particular third world travel. If there has been recent travel, then enquire about:
  - Dates of travel
  - Locations visited
  - Reason for travel
  - Type of accommodation
  - Ask about any illnesses whilst abroad or medical care
  - Travel vaccines and malaria prophylaxis/mosquito prevention if appropriate
  - Activities whilst abroad, e.g. eating, sexual contact, fresh water swimming

Medical history

- Any other medical condition or history of fever.

Family history

- Ask about health conditions affecting the family.

Drug history

- Use of anti-pyretics or antibiotic treatments.

Social history

- Smoking and alcohol intake
- Other unwell contacts

Interpretation and use of information gathered

- Differential diagnosis for this case:
  - Malaria
  - Respiratory tract infection e.g. influenza
  - Viral illness e.g. EBV and CMV
  - Dengue
  - Typhoid fever
  - Schistosomiasis
  - HIV seroconversion

Discussion related to the case

What is your most likely diagnosis and why?

- Malaria. My reasons for this are the combination of:
  - fever
  - multiple mosquito bites
  - history of travel to areas endemic for malaria
  - lack of antimalarials during his holiday

What do you know about malaria?

- Malaria is an infection that is commonly found in Africa, Asia, Central and South America.

- It is caused by an infection with the parasite *Plasmodium* – four types: *falciparum, vivax, ovale, malariae.*
- Transmission occurs via bites from infected female *Anopheles mosquitoes.*
- The parasite infects red blood cells and causes haemolysis.
- Malaria from Africa can be potentially very serious.
- Symptoms usually occur 1 to 4 weeks after becoming infected.
- Conditions such as sickle-cell disease, thalassaemia and G6PD deficiency provide some protection to the individual from the development of malaria.

What are the complications of malaria?

- Acidosis
- Hypoglycaemia
- Severe anaemia
- Shock
- Hepatic failure
- Renal failure
- Glomerulonephritis (*malariae strain*)
- Haemoglobinuria
- Cerebral oedema and coma (*falciparum strain*)
- Pulmonary oedema and respiratory distress (*falciparum strain*)

How would you diagnose malaria?

- Serology to detect malaria antigen.
- Repeated microscopy of thick and thin blood films – the disease is unlikely if there are three negative slides in 72 hours.

How would you treat malaria?

(a) Drug treatment

- Treatment depends on the type of malaria. Drug resistance is an increasing problem.
- *P. vivax, ovale* and *malariae* can usually be treated on an outpatient basis. Chloroquine or primaquine are often used.
- All patients with *P. falciparum* must be initially admitted to hospital owing to the possibility of rapid deterioration as the parasite replicates quickly.
- *P. falciparum* is resistant to chloroquine. Options incude quinine and doxycycline, co-artem (artemether and lumefantrine) or Malarone (atovaquone and proguanil).

(b) Severe malaria

- Antipyretics
- Intravenous fluids if dehydrated
- Intravenous glucose if hypoglycaemic
- Exchange transfusion if very high levels of parasites are found or complications develop
- ITU admission is needed if complications such as acidosis or cerebral or pulmonary oedema occur

Tell me about drug prophylaxis of malaria

- Infection can still occur with any of the recommended drugs.
- For areas with widespread chloroquine resistance, prophylaxis is with mefloquin, doxycycline or Malarone.
- For areas without chloroquine resistance, chloroquine and proguanil can be used.

I STATION 3 CARDIOVASCULAR AND NERVOUS SYSTEM

CARDIOVASCULAR SYSTEM

Mitral stenosis

Examine this patient's heart and describe your findings

The patient has a malar flush as well as a left thoracotomy scar. The pulse is irregularly irregular. The apex beat is tapping and not displaced. There is a left parasternal heave.* On auscultation of the mitral area there is a loud first heart sound (S1), opening snap, and mid-diastolic rumbling murmur heard loudest in held expiration in the left lateral position. The patient is clinically not in heart failure [the JVP is normal, no sacral/ankle swelling, and no basal crepitations in the lungs].

This patient has mitral stenosis.

*Indicates RVH, which may occur with pulmonary hypertension (in which you would find a raised JVP, loud P2 and RVH).

What other conditions give rise to a diastolic murmur?

- Aortic regurgitation – early diastolic murmur lower left sternal edge
- ASD – mid-diastolic murmur loudest in tricuspid area and fixed wide splitting of second heart sound
- Pulmonary regurgitation – early diastolic murmur at left sternal edge

What are the causes of mitral stenosis?

- Rheumatic fever in 50%
- Calcification
- Carcinoid
- Autoimmune conditions, e.g. RA
- Congenital

How would you assess the severity of mitral stenosis?

- Presence of pulmonary hypertension (described above)
- Duration of diastolic murmur is directly proportional to the severity of mitral stenosis

What complications can occur in this condition?

- Left atrial dilatation leading to AF
- Mural thrombus formation and embolization causing TIA/CVA
- Pulmonary hypertension
- Left heart failure leading to pulmonary oedema and haemoptysis
- CCF due to right heart failure (leading to ascites, hepatomegaly and tricuspid regurgitation)

What are the causes of AF?

Cardiac

- Ischaemic heart disease
- Mitral valve disease
- Hypertension
- Cardiomyopathies
- Myocarditis
- Atrial tumour

Infective

- Rheumatic fever
- Endocarditis
- Pneumonia

Endocrine

- Thyrotoxicosis

Drugs

- Alcohol or caffeine
- Digoxin
- Levothyroxine

Respiratory

- PE
- Lung malignancy

What do you know about the CHADS scoring system?

The CHADS2 scoring system predicts the risk of patients developing stroke in those with non-rheumatic AF. Tables 6 and 7 below demonstrate how the scoring system works and the probability of developing stroke.

Table 6 CHADS2 scoring system

	Medical condition	Score
C	CCF	1
H	Hypertension (BP > 140/90 mmHg)	1
A	Age at least 75 years	1
D	Diabetes mellitus	1
S 2	Past stroke or TIA	2

How would you determine which patients should be anticoagulated?

Table 7 CHADS2 scoring and the decision to treat

CHADS2 Score	Risk of stroke	Treatment
0	Low	None or aspirin
1	Moderate	Aspirin or oral anticoagulation
2	Moderate–high	Oral anticoagulation

Tell me about another useful scoring system for patients with AF

The CHA_2DS_2-VASc (Table 8) is a more detailed version of the CHADS2 scoring system, taking account of other risk factors for stroke.

Table 8 CHA_2DS_2-VASc scoring system

	Medical condition	Score
C	CCF	1
H	Hypertension (BP > 140/90 mmHg)	1
A 2	Age > 75 years	2
D	Diabetes mellitus	1
S 2	Past stroke or TIA	2
V	Vascular disease (e.g. peripheral artery disease, MI, aortic plaque)	1
A	Age 65–74	1
Sc	Sex category (female)	1

The risk of developing stroke and the need for treatment using CHA_2DS_2-VASc can also be followed from Table 7. The European Society of Cardiology does prefer anticoagulation for risk scores of ≥ 1. This is because they consider the risk–benefit ratio to have shifted in response to the use of newer anticoagulants (e.g. dabigatran), which are considered safer than warfarin.

What are the treatments for AF?

- The treatments are rhythm control or rate control (Table 9).
- Electrical or pharmacological cardioversion is used to achieve sinus rhythm (rhythm control).
- Pharmacological agents are used to achieve rate control.

Table 9 Rhythm versus rate control for AF

Rhythm (electrical or chemical)	Rate (e.g. digoxin, verapamil, β-blockers)
Age < 65	Age > 65
New-onset AF	Coronary heart disease
Symptomatic patients, e.g. chest pain, lightheadedness, heart failure	Unsuitable for cardioversion, e.g. chronic AF, ongoing reversible causes
Secondary to treated or corrected precipitant	Contraindication to antiarrhythmics

Note:

- Cardioversion should be carried out ideally within 24 hours of the onset of AF (due to the risk of left atrial appendage thrombus formation, which can be present in up to 15% of patients within this time). Cardioversion (electrical or drug) should be avoided after this time without adequate anticoagulation (unless one excludes atrial thrombus with TOE first).
- Chemical treatments for cardioversion include amiodarone and sotolol.
- Anticoagulation – vitamin K antagonists (warfarin, acenocoumarol, phenindione) inhibit synthesis of vitamin K-dependent clotting factors. Their action can be reversed by vitamin K. The most widely used among these, warfarin, decreases the risk of ischaemic stroke by over two-thirds. Aspirin reduces it by over one-fifth. One needs to balance the risk of stroke with the risk of bleeding (particularly in patients over 75 years old or those with uncontrolled hypertension or a history of bleeding) on this treatment.
- Newer anticoagulation agents are likely to become more available, e.g. dabigatran and apixaban.

Tell me what you know about the newly available oral anticoagulants

- Dabigatran etexilate: inhibits thrombin synthesis. Licensed for prophylaxis of VTE in adults with non-valvular AF and associated risk factors or after hip or knee replacement surgery. It does not require monitoring and has equivalent efficacy to warfarin in preventing VTE, but there is no available antidote and it is substantially more expensive. Dosage is twice daily.
- Rivaroxaban: inhibits factor Xa synthesis. Licensed for prophylaxis of VTE in adults after hip or knee replacement surgery. It does not require monitoring and has equivalent efficacy to warfarin in preventing VTE, but there is no available antidote and it is substantially more expensive. Dosage is once daily. Its role in prevention of VTE in AF is currently being reviewed.

What investigations would you perform in a patient with mitral stenosis?

- ECG – P mitrale suggested by bifid P waves
- CXR
  - enlarged left atrium
  - upper lobe diversion of blood flow
  - right atrial enlargement

- Echocardiography – two-dimensional echocardiography identifies mural thrombus, atrial enlargement and severity of stenosis
- Doppler studies – to assess pressure gradients/coronary arteries
- Catheterization if ischaemic heart disease is suspected

What are the treatment options for such patients?

Conservative

- In mild disease simple follow-up

Medical

- Anticoagulation – for AF, embolization, left atrial enlargement, moderate stenosis
- Treat complications (listed above)
- Endocarditis prophylaxis – see NICE guideline on antimicrobial prophylaxis against infective endocarditis

Surgical

- Indications
  - haemoptysis
  - pulmonary hypertension
  - recurrent embolization
- Methods – valvotomy (closed and balloon, also open method), valve replacement

What do you know about antibiotic prophylaxis for endocarditis?

- Adults and children with various conditions are at risk of developing infective endocarditis, including those with:
  - structural congenital heart disease (except for ASD, repaired VSD, PDA and endothelialized closure devices)
  - acquired valvular heart disease
  - valve replacements
  - previous infective endocarditis
  - HOCM
- Use of antibiotics:
  - NICE released a guideline on prophylaxis of endocarditis in 2008 (NICE guideline CG064; London: NICE, 2008. Available at: http://www.guidance.nice.org.uk/CG064. Accessed 14 February 2012)

> - Antibiotic prophylaxis is not recommended for any dental, gastrointestinal or respiratory tract procedure.
> - There is no evidence that chlorhexidine reduces the risk of infective endocarditis in people undergoing dental procedures.
> - People at risk of developing infective endocarditis should have all episodes of infection investigated and treated promptly.

- Patients at risk of developing endocarditis who are due to have a gastrointestinal or genitourinary procedure at a suspected infection site should be given antibiotics that cover organisms that cause endocarditis.
- The most common organisms that cause endocarditis are:
  - viridans streptococci (48%)
  - staphylococci (30%)
  - enterococci (10%)
  - haemolytic streptococci (4%)
  - pneumococci (1%).

Patient advice

- Patients at risk of infective endocarditis should be informed of the risks and benefits of having interventional procedures and receiving antibiotic prophylaxis. They should be told why routine antibiotic prophylaxis is not recommended, which symptoms of infective endocarditis to look out for and when to seek medical advice. They should also be advised to ensure good oral health.

Mitral regurgitation

Examine this patient's heart and describe your findings

On examination, the pulse is regular and jerky. The apex beat is displaced (describe its location) and thrusting. There is a left parasternal heave and systolic thrill. The first heart sound is soft and there is a third heart sound. A pansystolic murmur is heard at the apex and radiates to the axillary region; this is heard loudest in held expiration with the patient in the left lateral position. There are no clinical signs of heart failure or pulmonary hypertension.

The patient has mitral regurgitation.

What might this murmur be confused with?

- VSD
- Tricuspid regurgitation
- Mitral valve prolapse

What are the causes of this condition?

- Rheumatic fever
- MI (usually presents acutely following ruptured chordae tendinae)
- Ischaemic heart disease
- Cardiomyopathy and left ventricular dilatation
- Autoimmune, e.g. rheumatoid arthritis
- Infective endocarditis
- Annular calcification

- Iatrogenic following mitral valve repair
- Genetic causes, e.g. Marfan's syndrome, Ehlers–Danlos syndrome, osteogenesis imperfecta

What investigations would you perform on this patient?

- ECG: P mitrale (less common than in mitral stenosis), LVH
- CXR: enlarged left ventricle, engorged pulmonary vessels
- Echocardiography: similar use to mitral stenosis, may help identify the cause
- Doppler studies: help determine valve gradients and pressures within the left ventricle and atrium/assess coronary arteries
- Catheterization: used in some circumstances

How would you manage patients with this condition?

Conservative

- Follow-up
- Endocarditis prophylaxis – see NICE guideline on antibiotic prophylaxis against infective endocarditis (p. 96)

Medical

- Treat complications (which are the same as for mitral stenosis)

Surgical

- If LVEF < 60%, consider surgery
- Options include valve repair or valve replacement (especially when severe regurgitation)

Mitral valve prolapse

This is also known as 'floppy mitral valve' and Barlow's syndrome.

Examine the heart and describe your findings

On examination the pulse is regular and of normal volume. The JVP is not raised. There are no thrills or heaves on palpation. On auscultation, there is a mid-systolic click in the apex area followed by a late systolic murmur. The murmur is accentuated by the Valsalva manoeuvre and by standing. Squatting decreases it. The patient is not clinically in heart failure.

The patient has mitral valve prolapse.

What is the underlying abnormality in this condition?

At least one mitral valve cusp is displaced into the left atrium during systole. This is the so-called 'floppy valve'.

How can this condition present?

- Usually asymptomatic and mild only
- Chest pain

- Syncope
- Palpitations – from arrhythmias including SVT
- Mitral regurgitation
- Embolization
- Sudden death

What are the causes?

Idiopathic

Connective tissue disorders

- SLE
- Osteogenesis imperfecta
- Ehlers–Danlos syndrome
- Marfan's syndrome

Cardiac

- Atrial myxoma
- Post mitral valve surgery
- Cardiomyopathies
- Ischaemic heart disease
- Myocarditis

Other

- Congenital
- Rheumatic fever

How would you investigate this patient?

- ECG: not often reliable, may show P mitrale, LVH and inverted T waves in the inferolateral leads
- CXR: often normal, may show left atrial enlargement
- Echocardiography (M mode): helps identify any mitral regurgitation, helps pick up posterior movement of mitral cusps in systole and identifies extent of left atrial and ventricular enlargement

What are the treatment options for these patients?

Conservative

- Reassurance for asymptomatic patients
- Endocarditis prophylaxis (see p. 96)

Medical

- Treat complications, e.g. antiarrhythmic for SVT, anticoagulants for embolization, β-blockers for arrhythmia

Surgery

- Valve repair/replacement if severe regurgitation present

Aortic stenosis

Examine this patient's heart and describe your findings

The patient has a slow-rising, small-volume pulse. The apex beat is heaving and undisplaced. There is a systolic thrill palpable over the aortic area. The second heart sound is soft, and there is an ejection click followed by an ejection systolic murmur radiating to the carotids. The murmur is heard loudest with the patient leaning forwards in held expiration. I would like to check the blood pressure for narrow pulse pressures. Clinically the patient is not in heart failure.

These findings are consistent with aortic stenosis.

What are the causes of this condition?

- Congenital – calcification, bicuspid valve
- Rheumatic heart disease
- Degenerative/calcific change – commonest in the elderly

How does this condition usually present?

- Coincidental finding (often at least moderate when symptoms develop)
- Exertional syncope
- Chest pain
- Breathlessness
- Heart failure (LVF more often than RVF)
- Sudden death

What is the differential diagnosis for an ejection systolic murmur?

- Aortic stenosis
- HOCM
- Pulmonary stenosis
- Supravalvular/subvalvular stenosis

How would you investigate this patient?

- ECG: if normal then there is unlikely to be significant aortic stenosis, changes may include LVH, conduction defects, P mitrale and left axis deviation
- CXR: can be normal, calcified aortic valve, post-stenotic aortic dilatation, cardiac enlargement
- Echocardiography: M mode is the gold standard for diagnosis
- Cardiac catheterization: to exclude coronary artery disease before valve replacement

Discussion the management of this condition

Conservative

- Avoid strenuous activity

Medical

- Treat complications (e.g. heart failure)
- Avoid nitrates (vasodilators can precipitate syncope)
- Endocarditis prophylaxis (page 96)

Surgical

- Indications for valve replacement:
  - gradient > 50 mmHg and symptomatic
  - LVF
  - LVH
  - VT
- Transcatheter aortic valve implantation is a new procedure being used in patients with severe disease who are not fit for an open valve replacement
- In children, valvuloplasty/valvotomy is the preferred choice
- Consider monitoring in less severe cases

Aortic regurgitation

Examine this patient's cardiovascular system and present your findings

The patient has a collapsing pulse which is bounding. There are visible arterial pulsations in the neck with a normal venous pressure (Corrigan's sign); there is also obvious head bobbing (De Musset's sign). The apex beat is displaced laterally to the anterior axillary line, seventh intercostal space. There is a high-pitched, early diastolic murmur at the lower left sternal edge heard loudest in held expiration with the patient leaning forward. There is also a diastolic murmur in the mitral area; in this context, this would be consistent with an Austin–Flint murmur. I would like to check the blood pressure to confirm the presence of a widened pulse pressure.

The patient has aortic regurgitation (AR).

Name some clinical signs, not already mentioned, that would suggest this diagnosis

- Hill's sign – BP in legs > BP in arms
- Quinke's sign – pulsation of nail bed
- Muller's sign – pulsation of uvula
- Traube's sign– loud systolic sounds over femoral arteries
- Duroziez's sign – diastolic murmur heard when femoral arteries compressed
- Third heart sound and loud P2 (suggesting pulmonary hypertension)
- Ejection systolic murmur (not necessarily in the presence of aortic stenosis)

What other signs might you look for clinically?

- Erythema marginatum, arthritis, fever and tachycardia (rheumatic fever*)
- Splinter haemorrhages, Roth's spots, microscopic haematuria (endocarditis*)
- Kyphosis, characteristic question mark posture, prominent abdomen (ankylosing spondylitis)
- Other signs of seronegative arthropathies, e.g. psoriatic

- Symmetrical small joint swelling (rheumatoid arthritis)
- Argyll Robertson pupils (syphilis)
- High arched palate, widened arm span (Marfan's syndrome)

*Commonest causes

Name some other possible causes of AR

Congenital	Acquired
Osteogenesis imperfecta	Hypertension
Bicuspid aortic valve	Leaking prosthetic valve
Hurler's syndrome	Aortic dissection
Coarctation of the aorta	

How would you investigate this patient?

- ECG – LVH with strain
- CXR – can be normal, sometimes calcification of valve present ± cardiomegaly
- Echocardiography – this confirms the lesion, may reveal underlying cause and assess severity
- Cardiac catheterization – helps determine left ventricular function, severity of aortic regurgitation as well as identify associated ischaemic heart disease

Discuss the management of this condition

Medical

- Endocarditis prophylaxis (see p. 96)
- Treat underlying cause
- Treat complications, e.g. heart failure (which is an advanced stage of AR)

Surgical

- Surgery will be required eventually in most cases.
- Timing of surgery is often a difficult decision. It is based on results of clinical status and investigations.
- Valve replacement is the preferred option (mechanical in the young and tissue valves in the elderly).

Pulmonary stenosis

Examine this patient's cardiac system and describe your findings

The pulse is of small volume. There is a prominent 'a' wave in the JVP (severe cases). On palpation there is a parasternal heave and systolic thrill in the pulmonary region. There is an ejection click along with split second heart sounds and soft P2 (pulmonary component). An ejection systolic murmur is heard in the pulmonary area with radiation to the left shoulder. This is best heard in held inspiration.

These findings are consistent with pulmonary hypertension.

Name some causes of pulmonary stenosis

- Congenital in most cases (associated with Fallot's tetralogy)
- Carcinoid syndrome – rare
- Rheumatic fever – rare

What are the main subtypes of pulmonary stenosis?

- Subvalvular
- Valvular
- Supravalvular

How would you investigate this patient?

- ECG – right ventricular hypertrophy
- CXR – oligaemic lung fields, enlarged pulmonary artery (due to post-stenotic dilatation)
- Doppler studies – reliable method of assessing severity of stenosis
- Echocardiography – identifies the location of stenosis. Also identifies RVH
- Catheterization – identifies the severity of stenosis

What are the treatment options in these patients?

Conservative

- Endocarditis prophylaxis (see p. 96)
- Mild cases have a good prognosis if untreated

Medical

- Treat complications (e.g. heart failure) and associated conditions (e.g. Fallot's tetralogy)

Surgical

- Balloon valvuloplasty is usually reserved for severe cases

Mixed mitral valve disease

Examine the heart and describe your findings

The patient has malar flush and a left thoracotomy scar. The pulse is regular at 80 beats/minute and of normal volume. Palpation reveals a thrusting, undisplaced apex beat, and there is a parasternal heave present. On auscultation there is a soft first heart sound, a pansystolic murmur and mid-diastolic rumbling murmur at the apex.

This patient has mixed mitral valve disease.

What do you think is the predominant valvular pathology?

The malar flush and undisplaced apex point towards mitral stenosis. However, the thrusting apex, soft first heart sound and pan-systolic murmur suggest mitral regurgitation, and I think that this is the predominant lesion. However, I think that an echocardiogram would resolve this question.

Mixed aortic valve disease

Examine this patient's heart and present your findings

Pulse is regular at 75 beats/minute and is of large volume. It is collapsing in nature. The venous pressure is normal. The apex beat is displaced laterally by 2 cm, in the sixth intercostal space. It is thrusting in nature and there is a systolic thrill. On auscultation there is a loud ejection systolic murmur heard loudest in the aortic area radiating to the carotids, along with an early diastolic murmur loudest at the lower left sternal edge. These murmurs are heard best with the patient leaning forwards in held expiration. I would like to check the blood pressure to confirm the pulse pressure.

This patient has mixed aortic valve disease.

The patient's blood pressure is 150/60 mmHg. What do you think is the dominant lesion?

The presence of a large volume/collapsing pulse, displaced/thrusting apex and widened pulse pressure suggest AR as the main lesion. However, I would like to perform echocardiography to confirm this.

Prosthetic heart valves

Examine this patient's heart and report your findings

The pulse is of normal volume, and the JVP is not raised. The patient has a vertical thoracotomy scar. There is a normal first heart sound and a metallic-sounding second sound with an ejection systolic murmur associated with a click heard loudest in the aortic region. There is no diastolic murmur and clinically this patient is not in heart failure and has no stigmata of endocarditis (offer to check eyes for Roth's spots, urine for microscopic haematuria and temperature chart for fever).

This patient has a prosthetic aortic valve with no clinical signs to suggest leakage or endocarditis.

What are the likely reasons this patient has a prosthetic valve?

- AR
- Aortic stenosis

What are the complications of prosthetic valves?

- Valve dehiscence
- Obstruction of valve due to thrombus
- Leakage due to tear/fracture
- Haemolysis at the valve
- Bacterial endocarditis (also a cause of leakage)
- Thromboembolism (anticoagulation for prosthetic valves)

What are the different types of heart valves?

Mechanical

- Require anticoagulation
- Most durable kind of valve
- Most appropriate in younger patients
- Metallic valves, e.g. ball cage, tilting disc and bileaflet

Biological

- Do not require anticoagulation
- Allografts, e.g. cadaveric
- Xenografts – porcine valves, pericardial valves (from the pericardial sac of cow/horse attached to a metal frame)

Absent radial pulse

Palpate this patient's upper limb pulses and describe your findings

The patient has an absent radial pulse on the left side. All other pulses are of normal volume, character and rhythm. I would like to check all the other pulses and the blood pressure in both arms.

What would be the causes of this abnormality?

- Congenital: Holt–Oram syndrome
- Iatrogénic: following arterial line, brachial artery catheterization, surgical tie off, Blalock–Taussig shunt (connects subclavian to pulmonary artery)
- AF: causing embolization
- Cervical rib
- Takayasu's disease

Fallot's tetralogy

Examine this patient and describe your key findings

The patient has clubbing. There is central cyanosis. A left parasternal heave is palpable along with a pulmonary systolic thrill. On auscultation there is an ejection systolic murmur heard loudest in the pulmonary region. The presence of a weak left radial pulse and thoracotomy scar suggest this patient has a Blalock–Taussig shunt.

These signs suggest a diagnosis of Fallot's tetralolgy.

What is a Blalock–Taussig shunt?

It is an anastomosis connecting the left subclavian artery with the left pulmonary artery. This is used very rarely nowadays as cardiopulmonary bypass allows for full correction of the defects.

What are the main features of Fallot's tetralogy?

- VSD
- RVH

- Pulmonary stenosis
- Over-riding aorta

What are the complications of Fallot's tetralogy?

- Endocarditis
- Paradoxical embolus
- Cerebral abscess
- Polycythaemia
- Eisenmenger's syndrome

What would be the most helpful investigations in patients with Fallot's tetralogy?

- CXR – oligaemic lung fields, boot-shaped heart and RVH
- Echocardiography – confirms the VSD and over-riding aorta. Doppler studies identify the pulmonary stenosis

What are the main treatments for Fallot's tetralogy?

- Total correction:
  - performed at an early age, commonest treatment nowadays
  - requires cardiopulmonary bypass
- Palliative shunts:
  - restores pulmonary blood flow
  - includes Blalock–Taussig shunt (connects subclavian to pulmonary artery), anastomosis from aorta to pulmonary artery (includes Potts' shunt, Waterson's shunt)

What is the prognosis for Fallot's tetralogy?

- 95% mortality prior to adulthood if uncorrected
- 90% survive into adulthood if corrected – the majority of these patients will have normal exercise tolerance

What are the main distinguishing features between this patient and one who has Eisenmeger's syndrome?

Inspection

- A thoracotomy scar is more likely in Fallot's tetralogy than in Eisenmenger's syndrome.

Palpation

- There is a pulmonary thrill in Fallot's tetralogy but not in Eisenmenger's syndrome.
- Pulses are weaker on the left side in Fallot's tetralogy than they are in Eisenmenger's syndrome.

Auscultation

- There is a loud pulmonary systolic murmur in Fallot's tetralogy, not present in Eisenmenger's syndrome.

CXR

- There are small pulmonary arteries in Fallot's tetralogy, large in Eisenmenger's syndrome.

Ventricular septal defect

Examine this patient's heart and describe your key findings

The patient's pulse is regular with normal JVP. The apex beat is minimally displaced laterally and there is a palpable systolic thrill over the precordium. There is a pansystolic murmur heard loudest at the lower left sternal edge with radiation to the mitral area. There is also a right ventricular heave and a second pulmonary heart sound.

This patient has VSD complicated by pulmonary hypertension.

Describe some associations of this condition

- Down's syndrome
- Turner's syndrome
- Fallot's tetralogy
- Post MI

What are the different subtypes of this condition and which is the commonest?

- Membranous – commonest type
- Muscular
- Infundibular
- Posterior

What investigations would you perform in such patients?

- ECG – may be normal with a small defect. If it is a large defect, then there will be LVH and RVH (related to pulmonary hypertension).
- CXR – again, normal with smaller defects. With larger defects, LVH and RVH. If there is pulmonary hypertension, there may also be enlarged central pulmonary vessels and oligaemic lung fields.
- Echocardiography/Doppler studies – reveal location of the VSD, pressures within the right ventricular chamber and the direction of shunting (with colour flow Doppler).
- Cardiac MRI – also useful in identifying and quantifying the shunt.

What are the complications of VSD?

Small VSD

- Infective endocarditis (also in large VSD)

Moderate–large VSD

- Pulmonary hypertension
- Eisenmenger's complex

- Aortic regurgitation
- CCF

What is the management of this condition?

Small VSDs

- Commonest type, usually asymptomatic and close spontaneously
- Antibiotic prophylaxis (endocarditis prevention; see p. 96)
- Surgery is not usually performed

Moderate–large VSD

- Surgical correction usually performed

Atrial septal defect

Examine this patient's heart and discuss your findings

The patient has a regular pulse, and JVP is normal. Apex beat is not displaced. There is a left parasternal heave. Auscultation reveals a fixed split second heart sound with an ejection systolic murmur heard loudest in the pulmonary region. There are no signs of pulmonary hypertension or heart failure.

The patient has ASD.

Discuss the different types of this condition

Secundum defect

- Accounts for 75% of ASDs
- Defect in the middle part of the atrial septum
- Usually presents in the third or fourth decades
- Increased chance of sinus nodal disease and AF

Primum defect

- 10–15% of ASDs
- Presents in childhood
- Defect in the lower part of the atrial septum
- More commonly associated with Down's syndrome
- Mitral and tricuspid regurgitation occur

Venosus defect

- 10–15% of ASDs
- Presents in infancy
- Location of defect near junction of superior (SVC) and inferior vena cava (IVC)

What are the complications of this condition?

- Pulmonary hypertension
- Eisenmeger's syndrome

- Infective endocarditis
- Paradoxical embolus
- AF
- Chest infections
- CCF

What investigations would you request in such a patient?

- ECG – right axis deviation in secundum defect and left axis deviation in primum defect
- CXR – enlarged pulmonary conus, right atrial and ventricular enlargement, clear lung fields, small aortic knuckle
- TOE and colour flow Doppler studies – identify the defect
- Contrast (or 'bubble') echocardiography – a relatively new technique in which a solution of agitated saline is injected and this can be seen on the echocardiogram to identify the ASD
- Other tests:
  - cardiac MRI
  - cardiac catheterization studies - help determine the size of the shunt

What is the management of this condition?

- Small ASDs may be left alone with monitoring.
- Surgery is indicated when pulmonary flow is 1.5 times > systemic flow.
- Surgery is contraindicated if Eisenmenger's syndrome has developed or if the patient is cyanotic.

Patent ductus arteriosus

Examine this patient's heart and describe your findings

The patient has a regular pulse which is collapsing in nature. The JVP is normal. There is a heaving apex beat and left parasternal heave. On auscultation there is a continuous 'machinery' murmur which is loudest in the left upper sternal margin. There is an absent second heart sound.

This patient has a PDA.

Describe the pathogenesis of this condition?

A PDA occurs when the ductus arteriosus fails to close and become the ligamentum arteriosum. Consequently, there is a shunting of blood from the aorta (distal to the left subclavian) into the pulmonary artery. This causes an increased flow of blood through the pulmonary circulation and left heart.

What are the complications?

- Heart failure
- Pulmonary hypertension
- Endocarditis
- Rupture of ductus
- Reversal of blood flow leading to cyanosis and clubbing (rare)

What other conditions may cause a continuous murmur and collapsing pulse?

- Mitral regurgitation and AR
- VSD and aortic regurgitation

Are there any other conditions causing a continuous murmur?

Yes: pulmonary arteriovenous fistula and venous hum

What investigations would you perform in this patient?

- CXR – shows increased pulmonary flow and enlarged pulmonary conus
- ECG – often normal
- Echocardiography/Doppler studies – identify the lesion, extent of LVH and reveals continuous pulmonary flow
- Cardiac catheterization – also establishes the shunt and its severity

What is the management of this condition?

- Prostaglandin inhibitors, e.g. indometacin – most effective in the first few weeks after birth
- Ligation and transection in other patients

Coarctation of the aorta

Examine this patient's heart and present your findings

The patient's upper body is better developed than the lower body. There are increased volumes in the radial and carotid pulses. The femoral arteries are of reduced volume and there is radiofemoral delay when palpating the pulses simultaneously. The JVP is normal. There are vigorous carotid pulsations in the neck. On palpation the apex beat is heaving and there is a thrill in the suprasternal notch. A systolic murmur is heard over the precordium which can be heard in the back and in the second intercostals space anteriorly. I would also like to check the blood pressures in the arms and legs.

These findings are consistent with coarctation of the aorta.

What associated conditions would you look out for?

- Turner's syndrome
- Marfan's syndrome
- PDA
- VSD
- Mitral valve disease

What is the significance of checking the blood pressure in the arms and legs?

In coarctation of the aorta there is hypertension in the upper body with a lower blood pressure in the legs.

Discuss what happens in this condition

- This is a congenital condition, commoner in males, in which the aorta is narrowed (usually sited near the ligamentum arteriosum).
- Blood is diverted to the lower body via a collateral circulation in the periscapular and intercostal arteries.
- There is upper body hypertension as a result of the coarctation.
- There are different forms of coarctation of the aorta according to the anatomical location of the defect as well as the extent of constriction (ranges from mild obstruction up to atresia).
- Sometimes the coarctation occurs proximal to the left subclavian artery which results in lower blood pressure in the left arm than in the right arm.

What are the complications of this condition?

- Aortic dissection
- Hypertension
- Premature ischaemic heart disease and stroke
- Aortic stenosis (due to associated bicuspid aortic valve in 50%)
- Heart failure
- Lower limb claudication
- Endocarditis
- Subarachnoid haemorrhage (from associated berry aneursyms)

What investigations would you perform on this patient?

- CXR – '3' sign over the aortic knuckle (due to dilatation of the aorta with indentation at the site of coarctation), also rib notching (due to collaterals which erode the undersurface of the ribs)
- ECG – LVH
- Echocardiography – identifies the coarctation
- Doppler studies – confirm the discrepancy in blood pressure between upper and lower body
- MRI – helpful in identifying the lesion, commonly used
- Catheterization and angiography – not always required

How would you manage this group of patients?

- Significant coarctation corrected early by balloon dilatation or surgical correction
- Surgical correction consists of resection of the coarctation with end-to-end anastomosis of the aorta
- Stenting of the lesion – still in the experimental stages
- Treat hypertension
- Endocarditis prophylaxis if uncorrected or there is an associated valve lesion, e.g. bicuspid aortic valve

What is the prognosis of this condition?

- Mortality is 75% by age 50 if the condition is not treated.
- The prognosis is better the earlier the coarctation is repaired (> 80% survival after 25 years if repaired in childhood, 75% survival after 25 years if repaired between ages 20 and 40, and 50% survival after 15 years if repaired after age 40).

Eisenmenger's syndrome

Examine this patient's heart

The pulse rate is normal with regular volume. This patient has clubbing of the fingers and central cyanosis. There is a large 'a' wave in the JVP. On palpation there is a left parasternal heave and palpable second heart sound (P2). There is a loud, fixed/split second sound; in the pulmonary region, there is an ejection click and an early diastolic murmur (Graham Steell murmur). The patient also has a loud pansystolic murmur heard loudest in the tricuspid region and accompanied by a 'v' wave in the JVP.

These findings are consistent with Eisenmenger's syndrome due to an ASD with signs of significant pulmonary hypertension.

What is Eisenmenger's syndrome?

This is a cyanotic heart disease occurring when pulmonary hypertension leads to a reversed or bidirectional shunt developing. The shunt can occur at atrial, arterial or ventricular level. When pulmonary pressure is greater than systemic pressure, the result is a right-to-left shunt. Deoxygenated blood bypasses the pulmonary circulation, which causes cyanosis and clubbing of the fingers.

Give some examples of the conditions that lead to Eisenmenger's syndrome

- Atrial level – ASD
- Arterial level – PDA
- Ventricular level – VSD

What complications might develop in this patient?

- Right heart failure
- Pulmonary infarction
- Arrhythmias
- Endocarditis
- Cerebral abscess
- Paradoxical embolus
- Abnormal clotting (bleeding or thrombosis formation)
- In pregnancy: high rate of spontaneous abortion and high mortality rate in mothers if there is underlying VSD (therefore pregnancy is not advised in these patients)

What investigations would you perform?

- CXR – dilated pulmonary trunk and narrowing of peripheral pulmonary vessels, right ventricular hypertrophy in ASD
- ECG – P pulmonale, LVH/right ventricular hypertrophy
- Echocardiography – identifies the shunt and pulmonary hypertension, assesses ventricular function

How would you manage this patient?

In most cases, correction of the underlying defect will not treat the condition once Eisenmenger's syndrome has set in.

Conservative

- Treat complications (e.g. heart failure, arrhythmia)
- Phlebotomy for polycythaemia
- Oxygen
- Prostaglandin analogues

Heart–lung transplant

- *High-risk* procedure, limited donor availability

What is the prognosis of this condition?

- Most patients die between the ages of 20 and 40.

Hypertrophic obstructive cardiomyopathy

Examine this patient's heart

The pulse is regular but jerky in character with normal volume. There is a prominent 'a' wave in the JVP. On palpation there is a double apical impulse; a systolic thrill at the left sternal border can be felt. Auscultation reveals a fourth heart sound and an ejection systolic murmur over the left third intercostal space; this is accentuated by getting the patient to stand (increases venous return). The murmur is decreased by getting the patient to squat (reduces venous return); it radiates to the aortic region but not to the carotids. There is also a pansystolic murmur at the apex with radiation to the axilla.

These findings are consistent with HOCM. I would like to confirm this with echocardiography.

How would echocardiography help?

An echocardiogram would help confirm the diagnosis. Classic findings include asymmetrical septal hypertrophy, reduced end-diastolic volume and systolic anterior motion of mitral valve.

How might this patient have presented?

Most patients are asymptomatic but modes of presentation are:

- AF
- heart failure
- arrhythmia
- embolization
- endocarditis
- can also present with sudden death

Briefly discuss the inheritance of this condition

HOCM usually follows an autosomal dominant pattern of inheritance. A range of mutations have been discovered coding for myofibrillary proteins.

How common is this condition and what is the risk of sudden death?

HOCM has an adult prevalence of 1 in 500, with an equal male : female preponderance. Patients have a 5% risk of sudden death per year.

What investigations would you like to perform in this patient?

- CXR – may be normal, may show left atrial/ventricular enlargement
- ECG – normal in 25% of patients. May show AF, ST depression/T wave changes, LVH or left axis deviation
- Echocardiography – discussed above
- Cardiac catheterization – assesses LVF
- Treadmill testing – if there are symptoms of angina (present in 25% of patients)
- Angiography – useful if trying to rule out ischaemic heart disease

How would you manage this patient?

Supportive

- Genetic counselling for patients and families
- Support groups
- Endocarditis prevention (see p. 96)

Medical

- Treat complications e.g. amiodarone for AF
- β-blockers (e.g. propranolol)
- Calcium channel blockers (e.g. verapamil)

Surgical

- Dual chamber pacing
- Septal ablation (chemical with alcohol, or surgical with myomectomy)

Dextrocardia

Examine this patient's heart

The pulse is of regular rate and good volume. The JVP appears normal. I am unable to detect an apex beat on the left side on palpation; however, I can elicit this on the right-hand side in the fifth intercostal space, mid-clavicular line. There are also corresponding heart sounds on the right-hand side. I would also like to examine the abdomen to detect the position of the liver. Lung fields are clear. I would like to perform a CXR.

The patient has dextrocardia.

Why would you like to perform a CXR?

- To confirm the diagnosis and to look for a gastric air bubble on the right side. I would also like to look for signs of bronchiectasis which would be consistent with Kartagener's syndrome.

What is Kartagener's syndrome?

- This is a congenital condition characterized by a disorder in cilial motility.
- Clinically, the patient has situs inversus/dextrocardia, bronchiectasis, disorders of sinuses and infertility.

What is the significance of dextrocardia with situs inversus?

- If this is the case, then the likelihood is that the patient has an underling cardiac malformation e.g. Turner's syndrome.

Marfan's syndrome

Examine this patient's heart and discuss your findings

On inspection the patient is tall and has disproportionately long limbs compared with his trunk. There are small papules in the neck (Miecher's elastoma). His arm span is greater than his height. There is pectus excavatum and kyphoscoliosis. There is flickering of the iris. The patient has a regular pulse which is bounding and collapsing in nature. The JVP is normal. Vigorous carotid pulsations are seen in the neck. The apex beat is displaced laterally [state location]. On auscultation there is an early diastolic murmur heard loudest at the lower left sternal edge and in held expiration with the patient leaning forwards. I would like to check the blood pressure to confirm the presence of a widened pulse pressure.

The patient has AR with signs of Marfan's syndrome, although I would like to conduct a full examination to confirm this.

What other signs would you be looking for?

Cardiac

- AR
- Aortic aneurysm
- Coarctation of the aorta
- Mitral valve prolapse
- Endocarditis
- Aortic dissection

Eye

- Myopia
- Upward lens dislocation
- Blue sclerae
- Retinal detachment
- Glaucoma

Chest

- Pectus excavatum
- Spontaneous pneumothorax
- Emphysema
- Fibrosis
- Bronchiectasis

Musculoskeletal

- Hypermobility and laxity of joints

Other

- High arched palate
- Abdominal hernias

How is this condition inherited?

Inheritance is autosomal dominant causing defects in the fibrillin gene, which is on the long arm of chromosome 15.

What is the main differential diagnosis?

- Homocystinuria

What are the distinguishing features between these conditions?

- Upwards lens dislocation in Marfan's syndrome, downwards in homocystinuria
- More likely to have learning disability in homocystinuria
- Presence of homocystine in the urine using the cyanide–nitroprusside test

What is the prognosis of patients with Marfan's syndrome?

- There is a high incidence of cardiac complications causing most deaths in these patients.

How would you follow up and manage these patients?

- Regular echocardiography (especially for signs of aortic root dilatation)
- Early use of β-blockers to help reduce the progression of aortic root dilatation and there is also evidence that it decreases incidence of aortic rupture
- Ophthalmology referral
- Genetic counselling
- Treat other complications

Congestive cardiac failure

Examine this patient's heart and discuss your findings

The patient is dyspnoeic at rest. The pulse is regular with a normal rate and good volume. The JVP is elevated to 5 cm. The apex beat is displaced to the seventh intercostal space, anterior axillary line. There is a right ventricular heave present.

Auscultation reveals a third heart sound with no murmurs. There are crepitations in the lung bases and pitting oedema in the ankles up to the mid-shins. There are no stigmata of endocarditis. I would like to check for hepatomegaly and examine the blood pressure.

This patient has signs of CCF with no obvious cause.

What are the causes?

- Commonly ischaemic heart disease

Other cardiac causes

- Valvular heart disease
- Cardiomyopathy
- Endocarditis
- Hypertension
- Arrhythmia
- Congenital heart disease e.g. Fallot's tetralogy, septal defects, etc.

Chest

- PE
- Cor pulmonale

Drugs

- Alcohol
- Chemotherapeutic agents
- Cocaine

Other

- Anaemia
- Thyroid disease
- Paget's disease
- Burns
- Amyloidosis
- Sarcoidosis

How would you investigate this patient?

- Bloods – U&E, FBC, bone profile, TFTs, LFTs
- CXR – cardiomegaly, upper lobe diversion, bibasal effusion, Kerley B lines
- ECG – may reveal underlying cause, e.g. old infarct, AF, hypertrophy, 24-hour ECG if arrhythmia is suspected
- Echocardiography – identifies reduced ejection fraction, valvular heart diseases, cardiomyopthy, systolic/diastolic dysfunction
- Exercise testing – for signs of coronary heart disease
- Coronary angiography – for underlying ischaemic heart disease

How would you treat patients with chronic heart failure?

See Figure 3.

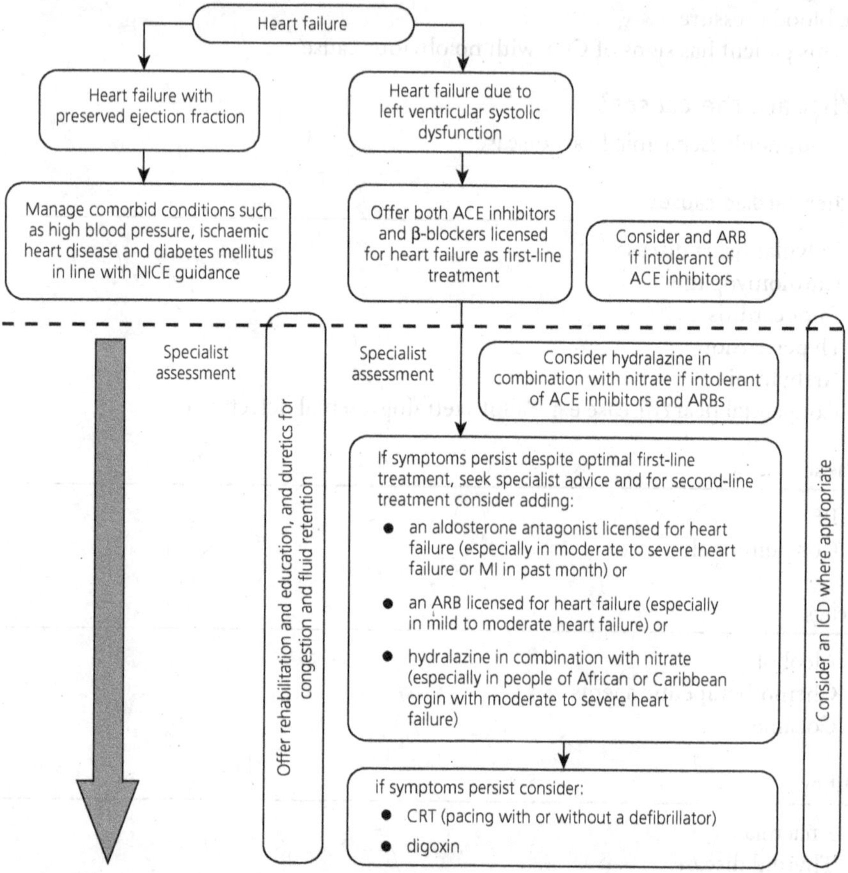

Figure 3 Treatment for chronic heart failure. Reproduced with permission of the National Institute for Health and Clinical Excellence from *Chronic heart failure: management of chronic heart failure in adults in primary and secondary care*, NICE guideline CG108. London: NICE; 2010. http://guidance.nice.org.uk/CG108 (accessed February 2012).

PERIPHERAL NERVOUS SYSTEM

Parkinson's disease (PD) and tremor

Examine this patient's hand and describe your findings

The patient has a resting pill rolling tremor of the left hand at approximately 4 Hz. This is worse at rest and relieved when moving the hand. I note the patient has mask-like facies. Examination of the upper limbs reveals cogwheel rigidity of the arms. I would also like to examine for a shuffling, festinating gait.

These signs are consistent with Parkinson's disease

Discuss some additional examination findings in a patient with PD

Signs are often asymmetrical.

Face

- Drooling of saliva
- Positive glabellar tap
- Blepharoclonus (tremor of the eyelids seen during gentle closure of the eyes)
- Head/jaw tremor

Upper limbs

- Lead pipe rigidity of the elbow
- Bradykinesia demonstrated by getting the patient to touch the thumb with each of the fingers

Gait

- Difficulty initiating movement
- Decreased arm swing

Speech

- Monotone
- Low volume

Handwriting

- Micrographia

What are the Parkinson plus syndromes?

These are a group of disorders characterized by features of Parkinson's disease as well as further features which make them more than idiopathic Parkinson's disease. Examples of these are:

- Shy–Drager syndrome: postural hypotension due to autonomic dysfunction
- Steele–Richardson syndrome (progressive supranuclear palsy): Parkinson's disease with supranuclear palsy resulting in defective vertical gaze

What are the main complications of Parkinson's disease?

- Falls
- Lewy body dementia
- Depression
- Drug side effects, e.g. on–off syndrome

Where does the pathology take place in Parkinson's disease?

Parkinson's disease is a neurodegenerative condition characterized by loss of dopaminergic neurons in the pars compacta region of the substantia nigra.

Explain the akinetic rigid syndromes and provide some examples

- The akinetic rigid syndromes are a form of movement disorder.
- They most commonly affect the extrapyramidal system and often include symptoms of rigidity, akinesia and tremor.
- Causes include:
  - Parkinson's disease (idiopathic)
  - Diffuse Lewy body disease
  - Corticobasal degeneration
  - Post-encephalitis
  - Cerebral anoxia, e.g. following trauma
  - Drugs: dopamine antagonists, MPTP (1-methyl-4-phenyl-1,2,3,6-tetrahydropyridine)
  - Multiple system atrophy
  - Progressive supranuclear palsy
  - Wilson's disease
  - Cerebrovascular disease

What are the treatment options for Parkinson's disease?

Supportive

- Multidisciplinary approach involving occupational therapists (walking aids, home equipment), physiotherapists, social worker, district nurses
- Support groups

Medical

- Dopamine agonists, e.g. cabergoline, ropinirole, bromocriptine
- Dopamine (levodopa) with dopa-decarboxylase inhibitor
- Catechol-O-methyltransferase (COMT), e.g. entacopone
- Monoamine oxidase inhibitors (MAOIs), e.g. selegeline

Surgical

- Subthalamic electrical stimulation

Name some different kinds of tremor

- **Resting tremor**: extrapyramidal disease, e.g. Parkinson's disease
- **Intention tremor**: cerebellar disease, accentuated by voluntary movements

- **Postural tremor:** brought on with fixed position (such as outstretched hand), e.g. benign essential tremor, alcohol, anxiety, thyrotoxicosis, drugs (lithium, tricyclics, sympathomimetics), syphilis
- **Physiological tremor:** causes similar to postural tremor

What do you know about benign essential tremor?

- This is a benign condition of unknown cause.
- It is more common in young adults but can occur at any age.
- There is often a family history.
- It is a postural tremor that is also present when performing movements.
- It tends to affect the arms, head and sometimes the legs.
- The condition is usually static but can cause significant distress to the patient.
- Common treatment would be a β-blocker.
- The tremor is relieved by alcohol. There is a risk of alcoholism as a result of the positive benefits attributed to alcohol.

What other kinds of involuntary movement disorders are there?

Apart from the akinetic rigid syndromes, the other group of movement disorders is the dyskinesias:

- **Essential tremor:** discussed above.
- **Chorea:** characterized by rapid movements of the hands or feet as if the patient is playing the piano. These occur for a brief period. Examples of such conditions include Huntington's and Sydenham's chorea, pregnancy and Wilson's diease.
- **Hemiballismus:** characterized by throwing movements on one side. Examples include infarcts of the contralateral subthalamic nucleus.
- **Myoclonus:** these are brief twitching movements of a muscle. Examples include Parkinson's disease, Creutzfeldt–Jakob disease (CJD), epilepsy, multiple sclerosis and hepatic failure.
- **Dystonia:** involves repetitive twitching or spasmodic movements of particular muscle groups. This includes writer's cramp, spasmodic torticollis, drug-induced (e.g. oculogyric crisis) and tardive dyskinesia.

Old polio

Examine this patient's legs

The patient has diffuse wasting in the right leg. Tone and power are also reduced on that side. Ankle and knee reflexes are absent. There are no fasciculations, sensation is intact and plantars are downgoing. The right leg is noticeably shorter than the left side. These findings are consistent with a lower motor neuron lesion affecting the anterior horn cells on the right side.

The most likely diagnosis is old polio.

Discuss the pathogenesis of this condition

- Polio is due to a virus called picornavirus.
- It affects the anterior horn cells of the spinal cord.

- Transmission usually occurs via the faeco-oral route but can also occur from saliva.
- It produces an initial paralytic illness, usually affecting one of the lower limbs in childhood, which then goes into a remission.
- Following remission, a slowly progressive weakness and wasting can develop. This usually involves the same muscle groups that were previously affected.

What else do you know about polio?

- It is commonest in developing countries.
- Pregnancy, recent tonsillectomy and vaccination are risk factors for developing the paralytic form of the illness.
- The illness may occur in a mild form that may pass unnoticed. The major form of the illness can present with paralysis.
- Treatment of acute polio is bed rest (helps prevent the paralytic form of the illness), analgesia and monitoring of vital capacity (to detect signs of respiratory muscle involvement). Ventilatory support and rehabilitation may also be required in some patients.

What vaccinations are there for prevention of polio?

- Inactivated (Salk) poliovirus: intramuscular route
- Live attenuated (Sabin) poliovirus: oral route

Abnormal gait

Examine these patients walking and discuss your findings

Case 1

There is a noticeable left-sided 'steppage' gait characterized by lifting the left foot high to avoid catching the toes on the ground due to foot drop.

The patient has weakness of tibialis anterior. This may be due to a lateral popliteal nerve lesion, old polio or Charcot–Marie–Tooth disease. It may also indicate nerve root compression at L4/5.

Case 2

This patient has an ataxic gait. The patient has a wide stance and is shaking as well as lunging. The patient appears to be falling to both sides as he is walking. I would like to conduct a full cerebellar examination.

This is a feature of cerebellar disease (vermis) or severe proprioceptive loss.

Case 3

This patient has a spastic gait. This is evidenced by the 'scissoring' movement (due to thigh adductor stiffness), slow movement and stiffness in the legs.

The causes could be congenital (e.g. hereditary spastic paraplegia, cerebral palsy) or acquired (multiple sclerosis, cord compression or space-occupying lesion).

Case 4

The patient has a hemiplegic gait. This is characterized by right-sided weakness and spasticity. The patient 'swings' the legs around as he is walking (due to the foot being in extension). The patient also has the arm held in flexion and adduction.

A hemiplegic gait is seen in an upper motor neuron lesion, usually due to a stroke.

Case 5

The feet stamp, the patient walks on a wide base and is watching the ground as he walks (due to loss of proprioception). The patient is unable to perform a tandem gait (walking heel to toe) and Romberg's test is positive (ataxia worsening by closing the eyes). I would like to complete my examination by testing for joint position and vibration sense as well as examining the cerebellar system (to rule this out as a possible cause of incoordination).

The patient has a sensory ataxia. Causes include: subacute combined degeneration of the cord, tabes dorsalis, Friedreich's ataxia and multiple sclerosis.

Proximal myopathy

Examine this patient's shoulders and hip muscles

The patient has weakness in his shoulder abductors and in extension of the hips. There is also difficulty in standing from the sitting position. There are no other neurological features of note in the upper limb. I would like to examine this patient's gait (looking for a waddling gait).

These findings are consistent with a proximal myopathy

Name some causes of proximal myopathy

Endocrine

- Cushing's syndrome
- Hyperthyroidism
- Hypothyroidism
- Conn's syndrome

Drugs

- Steroids
- Chloroquine
- Amiodarone
- Alcohol
- Lithium

Electrolyte imbalance

- Hypokalaemia
- Hypocalcaemia
- Hypomagnesaemia
- Hypophosophataemia

Congenital

- Mitochondrial myopathy
- Congenital myopathies e.g. myophosphorylase deficiency, muscular dystrophies

Rheumatological

- Polymyalgia rheumatica
- Osteomalacia
- Dermatomyositis/polymyositis

Infective

- Viral, e.g. influenza, coxsackievirus, HIV
- Bacterial, e.g. clostridial (*Clostridium welchii)*, staphylococcal and Lyme disease
- Parasitic, e.g. cysticercosis, toxoplasmosis

Other

- Renal failure
- Carcinomatous myopathy

Muscular dystrophy

Examine this patient's face and limbs

The patient has drooping of the mouth and wasting of the facial muscles with weakness in closing the eyes and in smiling. Abduction of the shoulders makes the superior margin of the scapula visible above the clavicles (anteriorly). When the patient is pushing against a wall with the arms extended, there is 'winging' of the scapula. There is also noticeable wasting of the shoulder girdle, pectoral and lower limb muscles. Of note, the patient has foot drop and weakness of eversion.

These findings are consistent with facioscapulohumeral muscular dystrophy.

Tell me about this condition

- It is autosomal dominant.
- It usually presents during childhood or early adult life.
- The gold standard in diagnosis is genetic testing. However, nerve conduction studies, muscle biopsy and electromyography (EMG) studies can also assist in diagnosis.
- Treatment revolves around a multidisciplinary approach focusing on addressing complications and dealing with social issues.
- Life expectancy is normal in most patients.

Briefly discuss the other kinds of muscular dystrophies

X-linked types

Becker's muscular dystrophy

- Onset is between 5 and 15 years, with patients wheelchair bound 20 years later.
- It is due to a mutation of the dystrophin gene.

Duchenne's muscular dystrophy

- Onset is at 3–4 years.
- It is also due to a mutation of the dystrophin gene.
- Patients develop hypertrophy of calf muscles/deltoids, lumbar lordosis and equinovarus deformity.
- There is the characteristic Gower's sign (using hands to 'climb up the legs' when standing up from the floor).
- Patients are confined to a wheelchair by age 10, lifespan is approximately 20 years.
- Unlike the muscular dystrophies mentioned above, this type affects cardiac muscle and leads to respiratory failure.

Autosomal recessive

- Childhood dystrophy – this is rare.
- Limb-girdle – onset in late teens to early twenties, predilection for shoulder or pelvic girdle initially, disability 20 years later. Patients with this condition have a normal life expectancy.

Autosomal dominant

- Myotonic dystrophy – see below
- Facioscapulohumeral dystrophy – discussed above
- Oculopharyngeal – tends to affect French Canadians
- Scapuloperoneal
- Ocular dystrophy

Myotonic dystrophy

Examine this patient's face and arms and present your findings

When shaking hands, the patient is slow to release his grip. He has myopathic facies (as in facioscapulohumeral dystrophy) with drooping of the mouth. He has frontal balding and a left-sided ptosis. There is wasting of the masseters, sternomastoids and temporalis muscles on the face. Upper limb reflexes are absent and there is weakness in the arm muscles with wasting of the distal muscle group. There is percussion myotonia in the thenar eminence. In addition, the dimple created by percussion is slow to fill. To complete my examination I would like to check for a red reflex (for cataracts), test his IQ and dipstick his urine for glucose.

This patient has myotonic dystrophy.

Tell me what you know about the epidemiology of this condition

- Autosomal dominant.
- The affected gene locus is located on chromosome 19.
- It affects males > females and tends to present in the twenties and thirties.
- Inheritance follows a pattern of anticipation (successive generations are affected more than preceding ones).
- Most patients' life expectancy is until middle age.

What other clinical features can patients present with?

- Oesophageal involvement causing dysphagia
- Distal muscle weakness, e.g. foot drop
- Cardiomyopathy and heart block
- Respiratory muscle involvement
- Cognitive decline and dementia
- Somnolence

How would you manage a patient with this condition?

Supportive

- Physiotherapy for weakness
- Podiatry, e.g. callipers for foot drop
- Occupational assessment
- Neurology follow-up

Medical

- Procanimide or phenytoin for advanced myotonia
- Treat complications, e.g. pacemaker for heart block

Genetic counselling

- For patients and relatives – the condition will be passed on to 50% of offspring

Tabes dorsalis

Examine this patient

The patient has a left-sided Argyll Robertson pupil with bilateral ptosis and frontal muscle wrinkling. Joint position and vibration sensation are lost in the legs. When squeezing the Achilles tendon there is loss of deep pain sensation and there are deformities of the knees (Charcot's joints). Tone and reflexes are also decreased in the legs. The patient has an ataxic 'steppage' gait and Romberg's test is positive.

These findings are consistent with tabes dorsalis.

What causes this condition and what part of the spinal cord is affected?

- It arises one to two decades following infection with *Treponema pallidum* (the agent causing syphilis). Tabes dorsalis is considered a tertiary form of syphilis.
- It involves degeneration of the dorsal columns of the spinal cord.

What are the other clinical features of the condition?

- 'Lightning' pains usually affecting the legs
- Constipation
- Foot ulcers
- Neurogenic bladder
- Loss of sensation in localized areas, e.g. testicular, thoracic area

What investigations would you perform in this patient?

Bloods

- VDRL test/TPHA – 75% sensitivity in tabes dorsalis
- FTA antibody
- False-positive FTA and TPHA antibodies appear in yaws and pinta

Other

- CSF – raised lymphocyte and protein counts
- MRI of the spinal cord – reveals enhancement of cranial nerves, meninges and spinal nerve roots

Please tell me about the blood tests for syphilis

- VDRL:
  - positive 3–4 weeks after primary infection
  - becomes negative 6 months after treatment
  - not specific for syphilis but useful to look at the titre in measuring disease activity and in screening
  - falling titre indicates successful treatment
  - rising titre suggests treatment failure or reinfection
  - a positive test reflects that an antibody produced by a patient with syphilis reacts with an extract of ox heart
- TPHA:
  - highly specific for *Treponema* antigens
  - patients with syphilis produce an antibody that agglutinates with sheep red blood cells coated with *T. pallidum*
- FTA-ABS:
  - also highly specific for *Treponema* antigens
  - the patient's serum antibodies attach to *T. pallidum* (which is fixed to a microscope slide)
  - this is highlighted with fluorescent anti-human immunoglobulins

How would you treat this patient?

Supportive

- Physiotherapy for ataxia
- Podiatry input for ulcers
- Self-catheterization for urinary incontinence

Medical

- IV penicillin
- Carbamazepine for lightning pains

Surgical

- Orthopaedic input for Charcot's joints

Apart from tabes dorsalis, what are the other manifestations of neurosyphilis?

Meningovascular syphilis

- It presents in the first decade following infection.
- It usually responds well to treatment.
- It can lead to a non-specific illness with headaches, confusion, seizures and signs of meningitis. Cranial nerve palsies and stroke are other complications. Optic atrophy often presents.

Syphilitic gumma

- Granulomas within the meninges presenting with focal neurological signs or convulsions

Generalized paralysis of the insane

- Usually presents 10–15 years following initial infection
- Associated with dementia, tremor, dysarthria and convulsions
- Treatment can reverse the condition in some cases or slow progression

Amyotrophy

- Rare form of neurosyphilis
- Characterized by degeneration of anterior horn cells

Peripheral neuropathy

Examine this patient's lower limb neurology

There is reduced symmetrical light touch and pin-prick sensations in a 'stocking' distribution of the legs. There is also impaired vibration sense and joint position sense. Ankle jerks are absent but other reflexes are intact. Tone and power are unremarkable. I would also like to check for similar findings in a 'glove' distribution of the upper limbs. I would also like to perform a urine dipstick for glucose and to check the eyes for jaundice and anaemia.

These findings are consistent with a peripheral neuropathy affecting the lower limbs.

What are the possible causes of a peripheral neuropathy?

- Diabetes mellitus
- Alcohol
- Toxic, e.g. lead, arsenic
- SACD; vitamin B_{12} deficiency
- Infection, e.g. leprosy, HIV, Lyme disease
- Iatrogenic, e.g. isoniazid, amiodarone, gold, metronidazole
- Autoimmune, e.g. rheumatoid arthritis, polyarteritis nodosa
- Neoplastic due to malignancy

- Renal failure
- Amyloidosis
- Porphyroid

What are the different types of neuropathy?

- **Mononeuropathy:** affecting a single nerve.
- **Mononeuritis multiplex:** occurs when more than one individual nerve is affected.
- **Polyneuropathy:** occurs when a large number of peripheral nerves are affected at the same time, usually in a symmetrical distribution, e.g. Guillain–Barré syndrome.

What are the causes of a mononeuritis multiplex?

- Diabetes
- Carcinoma
- Amyloidosis
- Sarcoidosis
- Lyme disease
- Leprosy
- PAN
- Rheumatoid arthritis
- SLE
- Churg–Strauss syndrome
- Sjögren's syndrome
- Wegener's granulomatosis
- HIV

What investigations would you carry out in a suspected case of neuropathy?

Tailor the investigations according to your differential diagnosis.

Bloods

- U&E, fasting glucose, autoantibody screen, vitamin B_{12} levels

Other

- Nerve conduction studies
- CXR to exclude malignancy or sarcoidosis

Discuss the spinal cord involvement in subacute combined degeneration of the cord (SACD)

- Dorsal column involvement is a hallmark of SACD.
- In the latter part of disease progression, the pyramidal tracts are affected. This can lead to pyramidal signs and spastic paraparesis.

What are the other clinical features of SACD?

- Anaemia
- Optic atrophy
- Retinal haemorrhage
- Extensor plantars and absent knee/ankle jerks
- Romberg's positive
- Cognitive impairment due to dementia

What are the causes of SACD?

- Anything causing vitamin B_{12} deficiency can lead to SACD.

Dietary

- Vegan diet
- Chronic alcoholics

Malabsorption

- Post gastrectomy
- Intrinsic factor deficiency:
  - pernicious anaemia
  - congenital deficiency
- Terminal ileal disease:
  - Crohn's disease
  - ileal resection
  - bacterial overgrowth
  - tropical sprue
  - fish tapeworm
- Coeliac disease
- Chronic pancreatitis
- Drugs, e.g. biguanides, potassium supplements

Metabolic causes

- Pregnancy
- Haemolysis
- Transcobalamin deficiency

What investigations would you perform to identify the cause of vitamin B_{12} deficiency?

Schilling test

Helps identify the cause (infrequently performed nowadays):

- Parenteral B_{12} is administered to saturate binding sites in plasma and liver.
- Following this radiolabelled oral B_{12} is given.
- Urinary excretion of radiolabelled B_{12} is measured. If normal, this suggests the cause of B_{12} deficiency is dietary.
- If the urinary radiolabelled B_{12} level is low, this suggests malabsorption:
  - In this case, combined oral intrinsic factor and radiolabelled B_{12} are then administered.
  - If this corrects the urinary excretion levels, this suggests the underlying deficiency is due to pernicious anaemia.
  - If combined intrinsic factor/radiolabelled B_{12} does not correct the urinary excretion levels, this suggests the patient has a malabsorption syndrome due to terminal ileal disease/bacterial overgrowth.

Bloods

- Autoantibodies to intrinsic factor and parietal cell (present in pernicious anaemia)

- Check folate, iron and vitamin D levels
- Coeliac screen

What is the treatment for vitamin B_{12} deficiency and how effective is it?

- Oral hydroxycobalamin or parenteral vitamin B_{12} can be used for patients with dietary deficiency.
- Parenteral vitamin B_{12} is required if it is due to malabsorption. This can improve the peripheral and sensory signs, but established motor signs are unlikely to respond.
- Administration of parenteral vitamin B_{12} is by three injections/week for 2 weeks then one injection every 3 months. Avoid use of folate until vitamin B_{12} levels are normal (to avoid precipitating SACD).

Ulnar nerve palsy

Examine this patient's arm and present your findings

On inspection the left hand shows small muscle wasting with sparing of the thenar eminence. There is wasting of the hypothenar eminence and dorsal guttering. The patient has a 'claw hand' appearance with hyperextension of the metacarpophalangeal and flexion of the fourth and fifth interphalangeal joints. There is loss of sensation in the medial one and a half aspect of the left hand and fingers on the dorsal and palmar surfaces.

This patient has a left ulnar nerve lesion.

What are the causes of an ulnar nerve palsy?

- Osteoarthritis at the elbow
- Cubitus valgus deformity
- Trauma from supracondylar fracture, elbow dislocation, wrist or hand injuries
- Occupational – due to leaning excessively on elbow (e.g. telephonist, desk jobs), frequent repetitive flexion/extension movements of the elbow (e.g. carpenter, bricklayer), excessive use of wrist and hands (e.g. builders, plumbers)
- Any cause of a mononeuritis multiplex (see p. 129)
- Space-occupying lesions e.g. neuromas and ganglions at the wrist level

Another patient with similar clinical signs has much less clawing and has a scar at the left elbow. Can you explain this?

- A more proximal lesion of the ulnar nerve has affected the flexor digitorum profundus.
- The deformity is less apparent in this case, i.e. there is less deformity. This is known as the 'ulnar paradox'.
- The scar represents a previous supracondylar fracture, which would have caused this.

Which muscles does the ulnar nerve supply?

- Flexor carpi ulnaris

- Flexors of the distal phalanx of fourth and fifth digits
- All intrinsic muscles of the hand except the thenar eminence

How would you test for ulnar weakness of the hand?

- Froment's sign – weakness in thumb adduction elicited by failure to grip a piece of paper between the thumb and index finger without flexing the thumb
- Weakness in flexion of fourth and fifth fingers
- Weakness in finger abduction and adduction

What is the differential diagnosis in this patient?

- C8/T1 lesion of the brachial plexus e.g. Pancoast's tumour, motor neuron disease
- Syringomyelia
- Polio
- Rheumatoid arthritis

Radial nerve palsy

Examine this patient's arm and present your findings

The patient has wrist drop. The elbow and fingers are in a flexed position and the forearm is pronated. There is weakness in finger and wrist extension and weakness in finger abduction and adduction, which resolves when placing the hand flat on a table. There is also a sensory loss over the dorsum of the thumb.

The patient has a radial nerve palsy.

What muscles does the radial nerve supply?

- Triceps
- Brachioradialis
- Supinator
- Wrist and finger extensors

What are the causes of a radial nerve palsy?

- Saturday night palsy – usually after consuming lots of alcohol and sleeping with the head lodged in the upper arm. The radial nerve compresses against the middle third of the humerus. This affects all muscle groups supplied by the radial nerve except for the triceps
- Trauma in the axillary portion of the radial nerve – humeral fracture, pressure effect from crutches, dislocated shoulder. Uniquely these injuries will affect the use of triceps with loss of elbow extension and triceps reflex
- Trauma to posterior cord of brachial plexus, e.g. stab wound
- Lead poisoning

How would you manage radial nerve palsy?

- Treat the underlying cause
- Radial nerve palsies usually resolve in several weeks
- Wrist splints are used to correct the wrist drop
- Physiotherapy

Carpel tunnel syndrome (median nerve palsy)

Examine this patient's hand and present your findings

The patient has wasting of the thenar eminence. Sensation is reduced in the lateral three and a half fingers. Power is reduced when testing for thumb abduction/ flexion and opposition. I would also like to check for Tinel's sign (percussion over the palmar surface of the wrist leading to paraesthesia in the median nerve distribution) and Phalen's sign (flexion of the wrist for 1 minute also produces symptoms in the hand due to compression of the median nerve at the carpel tunnel). I would like to examine the patient for underlying causes.

This patient has carpel tunnel syndrome.

What are the causes of this condition?

- Hypothyroidism
- Idiopathic
- Diabetes
- Acromegaly
- Pregnancy
- Rheumatoid arthritis
- Osteoarthritis
- Trauma – penetrating injury, wrist fracture
- Occupational, e.g. use of vibrating tools
- Tuberculosis
- Amyloidosis

What muscles does the median nerve supply?

Remember: LOAF

- **L**ateral two lumbricals
- **O**ppenens pollicus
- **A**bductor pollicus
- **F**lexor pollicus brevis

What investigations would you perform in this patient?

- Blood tests:
  - TFTs
  - FBG
  - OGTT (for suspected acromegaly)
  - RF
- Nerve conduction studies– reduced velocity in median nerve conduction

What treatments are available for this condition?

Conservative

- Wrist splints
- NSAIDs

Invasive

- Local steroid injection
- Surgical decompression

Common peroneal palsy

Examine the neurology of this patient's legs

On inspection the patient has wasting in the muscles of the right lateral leg (tibial and peroneal muscles) and there is a right-sided foot drop. There are no scars visible over the surface of the fibular head. There is decreased sensation over the lateral surface of the lower right leg and the dorsal surface of the right foot. There is a reduced power in eversion and dorsiflexion of the right foot and the patient has a 'steppage' gait. The reflexes are normal.

This patient has a right-sided common peroneal nerve palsy. I would like to investigate for an underlying cause.

What are the possible causes in this patient?

- Trauma to common peroneal nerve, e.g. at head of fibula from fracture
- Compression of nerve, e.g. from plasters
- Any cause of a mononeuritis multiplex (see p. 129 for causes)

Tell me about foot drop?

- Foot drop occurs when there is weakness of the anterior tibialis, which is responsible for dorsiflexion of the foot.
- This is supplied by the common peroneal nerve. Therefore, many of the causes of foot drop can be deduced by considering the anatomy of the innervation of the common peroneal nerve, in addition to any of the causes of mononeuritis multiplex and local muscle problems.
- Causes include:
  - weakness of anterior tibialis:
    - trauma
    - myositis
    - muscular dystrophy
  - common peroneal nerve pathology:
    - Charcot–Marie–Tooth disease
    - any cause of mononeuritis multiplex
  - sciatic nerve pathology
  - lumbosacral plexopathy
  - L4/L5 nerve root pathology:
    - herniated disc
    - tumour
  - spinal cord and brain pathology:
    - MS
    - tumour
    - vascular event

What tests would you perform in this patient?

- Blood tests looking for causes of mononeuritis multiplex
- Nerve conduction studies – will show peroneal nerve palsy
- Radiograph of fibula if a fracture is suspected

What treatments are available?

- Treat underlying cause, e.g. fracture
- Supportive footwear, e.g. calliper shoes

Guillain–Barré syndrome

This patient has developed weakness over the past 2 days. Please examine the face and arms

The patient has a bilateral lower motor neuron facial weakness. There is weakness in the upper limbs, more pronounced distally. There are absent supinator, biceps and triceps reflexes. Sensation is also affected symmetrically with a reduction in light touch in a glove distribution with impaired joint position sense. These features are consistent with an acute symmetrical polyneuropathy.

The main differential would be Guillain–Barré syndrome.

What other differentials would need to be considered?

- Infections such as botulism, diphtheria, polio, Lyme disease
- Motor neuron disease (does not produce sensory signs)
- Toxic causes such as organophosphate poisoning, thallium, arsenic
- Multiple sclerosis
- Porphyria
- Myasthenia gravis
- Myopathic disorders

What other clinical features are there in Guillain–Barré syndrome?

- Numbness and paraesthesia
- Autonomic dysfunction causing labile blood pressure, tachycardia
- Bulbar palsy
- Papilloedema
- Respiratory failure
- Ascending weakness and paralysis

What is Miller–Fisher syndrome?

- This a rare condition.
- In reverse order to Guillain–Barré syndrome, there is a descending weakness.
- It presents with a triad of opthalmoplegia, areflexia and ataxia.
- Treatment is the same as for Guillain–Barré syndrome (stated below).
- Prognosis is good, with most patients making a full recovery within 6 months.

How would you confirm that this patient has Guillain–Barré syndrome?

- Nerve conduction studies confirm demyelination.
- CSF shows increased protein levels.

What are the treatment options for Guillain–Barré syndrome?

Supportive

- Vital capacity, pulse and BP monitoring
- Blood gases
- Physiotherapy for weakness

Medical

- Plasmapheresis
- IV immunoglobulin

Invasive

- Mechanical
- Ventilation for respiratory failure

What is the prognosis for patients with Guillain–Barré syndrome?

- Most patients make a full recovery within a year of onset of the condition.
- 5% of patients are left with disability.
- The mortality rate is approximately 4%.

Wasting of the small muscles of the hand

Examine this patient's hands

The patient has wasting of the small muscles of the right hand. There is dorsal guttering and wasting of both thenar and hypothenar eminences. There are no other neurological features in the upper limbs. There is a right-sided Horner's syndrome characterized by ptosis, enopthalmos, miosis and anhydrosis. I would also like to examine the patient's chest and lymph nodes.

These findings indicate a lesion affecting C8/T1 at the brachial plexus, most likely a Pancoast's tumour.

What other causes are there for small muscle wasting of the hands?

Lesions affecting the C8/T1 nerve supply of the hands

- Syringomyelia
- MND
- Cord compression
- Polio

- Space-occupying lesion
- Cervical spondylosis (rare)
- Trauma to brachial plexus
- Charcot–Marie–Tooth disease
- Cervical rib
- Meningovascular syphilis
- Traumatic causes

Other causes

- Combined ulnar/median nerve palsy
- Disuse atrophy, e.g. from rheumatoid arthritis

Which of these causes are due to pathology at the brachial plexus level?

- Pancoast's tumour
- Cervical rib
- Traumatic causes

Charcot–Marie–Tooth disease (peroneal muscular atrophy)

Examine this patient's lower limbs and describe your findings

On inspection, the patient's legs have an 'inverted champagne bottle' appearance. This is characterized by distal muscle wasting of shins and calves, with sparing of the thigh muscles. There is a bilateral foot drop along with a pes cavus deformity of both feet and clawing of the toes. Power is decreased in dorsiflexion of both feet and in extension of the toes. Ankle reflexes and plantar responses are absent. Sensation is reduced to light touch in a stocking distribution. Upon examining the gait, there is a steppage gait (due to the foot drop). This patient has a motor sensory neuropathy.

This patient most likely has Charcot–Marie–Tooth disease.

Tell me about the inheritance of this disease

- Usually follows autosomal dominant inheritance.
- Autosomal recessive and sporadic cases of the disease do exist.

What are the clinical features

- Small muscle wasting of the hands (can create similar appearance in the upper limbs as lower limbs)
- Tremor of the upper limbs
- Palpable nerve thickening – lateral popliteal and ulnar nerves
- Kyphoscoliosis
- Respiratory muscle weakness
- Optic atrophy

What are the main types of this condition?

Hereditary motor sensory neuropathy type I

- Presents in childhood
- Deformities are usually marked
- It is due to a demyelinating neuropathy (with slowing of nerve conduction velocities)

Hereditary motor sensory neuropathy type II

- Later onset, usually teens but sometimes later
- Clinical features are less pronounced
- It is due to an axonal neuropathy

What investigations would you carry out in a suspected case of Charcot–Marie–Tooth disease?

- Nerve conduction studies – as above
- Nerve biopsy
- Genetic testing – useful for most types but not all

What is the management for Charcot–Marie–Tooth disease?

There are no specific treatments for this condition. Patients are advised to keep active and to avoid weight gain (to avoid tension on the joints). Surgical options are used when deformities are severe.

Friedreich's ataxia

Examine this patient's cerebellar system

The patient has dysarthric speech. The patient has dysdiadochokinesis and intention tremor in the upper limbs. In the lower limbs there is heel–shin ataxia. Tone is hypotonic in both limbs. There is nystagmus and the patient has an ataxic gait. I note pes cavus and scoliosis deformities on inspection. This patient has a combination of cerebellar signs as well as pes cavus and scoliosis.

These signs are consistent with Friedreich's ataxia.

What else would you like to examine for?

- Absent ankle jerks and extensor plantars
- Impaired joint position and vibration sense in the lower limbs (dorsal column involvement)
- The cardiovascular system for signs of HOCM
- Optic atrophy

What do you know about this condition?

- Friedreich's ataxia is a hereditary ataxia.
- It follows an autosomal recessive pattern of inheritance.
- Family members may have minor signs of the condition, e.g. pes cavus and absent ankle jerks.

- Patients present in childhood.
- There tends to be a worsening in signs leading to eventual disability.
- Patients usually survive no longer than into their fifth decade.

What other features might this condition present with?

- Learning disability
- Diabetes mellitus
- LVH and arrhythmia (due to HOCM)

Which parts of the brain and spinal cord are affected by this condition?

- Dorsal columns
- Corticospinal tracts
- Spinocerebellar tracts
- Purkinjee cells of the cerebellum
- Peripheral nervous system

What are the causes of acquired cerebellar disease

- Alcohol
- Drugs: phenytoin, solvent abuse, mercury
- Hypothyroidism
- Vascular – infarct, haemorrhage
- Demyelination, e.g. multiple sclerosis
- Infective – HIV, TB, abscess
- Neoplastic – space-occupying lesion, paraneoplastic syndromes

Myasthenia gravis

Examine this patient's face

The patient has a bilateral ptosis, expressionless facies, and generalized weakness in all facial muscles, which is reflected when getting the patient to smile and close the eyes. The ptosis is more pronounced upon sustained upwards gaze. There is diplopia when examining eye movements. The patient has nasal speech. The patient has evidence of a myopathic disease process with fatigability (increased ptosis with sustained upward gaze). I would like to examine the upper limbs for signs of proximal muscle weakness, checking the sensation and reflexes (normal sensation/reflexes fits with a myopathic disease process), and perform a Tensilon test.

These findings are consistent with myasthenia gravis.

What is a Tensilon test?

- An anticholinesterase drug called edrophonium is administered IV.
- This reverses myasthenic weakness for up to a few minutes.
- Eye movements are usually examined.
- An initial test dose (1–2 mg) is given to monitor any adverse effects followed by a bolus dose (5–10 mg).

What conditions is myasthenia gravis associated with?

- Thymoma
- SLE
- Thyroid disease
- Rheumatoid arthritis
- Pernicious anaemia
- Polymyositis
- Diabetes

What conditions precipitate myasthenic crisis?

- Stress
- Infection
- Drugs including streptomycin, gentamicin, quinine and D-penicillamine

What other clinical signs would you look for in this patient?

History

- Weakness worse towards the end of the day and worse as exercise progresses
- Problems with eating – swallowing, chewing, regurgitation

Examination

- Fatigability demonstrated with eye movements (described above), repetitive counting (bulbar weakness), repetitive proximal muscle movements in the shoulder and lower limb girdles
- Muscle wasting occurs late in the disease
- Respiratory muscle weakness – usually a sign of myasthenic crisis, requires ventilatory support and intensive care

What investigations would you perform?

- Edrophonium test – an acetylcholine esterase inhibitor is used to increase the concentration of acetylcholine at the motor end plate. This improves muscle strength
- Electromyography (EMG) – shows a decremental response to repeated impulses
- Acetylcholine receptor antibodies – found in 80% of patients
- Antibody screen to check for associated autoimmune disease
- Vital capacity to check lung function
- CT or MRI of the mediastinum to check for thymus enlargement

Why might rheumatoid arthritis be important in this patient?

- It is an associated autoimmune condition.
- D-penicillamine, used in rheumatoid arthritis, can cause myasthenia gravis.

How would you treat this patient?

Supportive

Adopt a multidisciplinary approach:

- Neurology follow-up

- Physiotherapy for weakness and mobility
- Occupational therapy assessments
- Support groups.

Medical

- Pyridostigmine (long-acting acetylcholinesterase)
- Immunosuppression – steroids and azathioprine sometimes used in combination
- Plasmapheresis (removes circulating acetylcholine receptor antibodies) – used in myasthenic crisis

Surgical

- Thymectomy for thymoma

What is Lambert–Eaton syndrome?

- This is a differential of myasthenia gravis.
- It is often associated with small cell bronchial carcinoma.
- It is due to defective release of acetylcholine at the neuromuscular junction with antibodies to calcium channels being present. It can present in a similar fashion to myasthenia gravis.
- Unlike myasthenia, EMG studies show an *increase* in amplitude with repetitive stimulation.
- Guanidine helps with the weakness.
- Pyridostigmine has no effect in this condition.

What are the causes of bilateral extraocular palsies?

- Myasthenia gravis
- Graves' disease
- Cavernous sinus pathology
- Kearns–Sayre syndrome
- Miller–Fisher syndrome (variant of Guillain–Barré syndrome)

Motor neuron disease (MND)

Examine this patient's upper limbs

The patient has diffuse muscle wasting of the arms as well as small muscle wasting of the hands. Fasciculations occur in most muscle groups. Power is decreased diffusely bilaterally. Reflexes are exaggerated in the biceps on the right and the triceps on the left. Sensation is intact.

I would like to complete my examination by examining the lower limbs and cranial nerves and checking for cerebellar signs.

The mixed upper and lower motor neuron signs within the same muscle groups, in the absence of any sensory loss, would be consistent with MND.

What one investigation would you wish to perform in this patient?

- I would like to perform MRI of the cervical spine to exclude cervical cord compression, which is the most important diagnosis to eliminate.

What do you know about MND?

- This is a degenerative condition affecting the anterior horn cells.
- It affects the upper and lower motor neurons in the brain and spinal cord.
- MND does not affect the sensory or cerebellar systems. It also does not affect the ocular muscles.
- It is a rare condition with a poor prognosis. Death usually occurs within 3 years of diagnosis.

Describe some of the other signs you might expect to find in this patient

- Often asymmetrical signs occur (as in this patient)
- Lower limbs – similar to upper limbs, may have extensor plantars and foot drop
- Bulbar involvement – dysarthria, dysphonia (nasal speech), wasting/fasciculation of tongue, palatal weakness
- Wasting of muscle groups supplied by the cranial nerves

What are the main complications of this condition?

- Gradual generalized weakness
- Nasal regurgitation of fluids
- Chest infections
- Respiratory muscle weakness causing shortness of breath

What are the various types of MND?

- Amyotrophic lateral sclerosis (commonest type)
- Progressive muscular atrophy
- Bulbar palsy
- Primary lateral sclerosis

What investigations would you perform in this patient?

- Mainly a clinical diagnosis
- EMG studies – may support the diagnosis and help exclude other treatable myopathies
- MRI – to exclude cervical cord compression

What are the treatment options for this patient?

- There is no cure currently available for MND
- Management involves a multidisciplinary team approach

Supportive

- Speech therapy for communication issues including electronic devices, monitoring of swallowing difficulties to help prevent aspiration (nasogastric/gastrostomy tubes in advanced cases)
- Physiotherapy for weakness, nursing care for disability
- Motor Neurone Disease Association

Medical

- Treat complications, e.g. cramps, contractures
- Riluzole (glutamic acid antagonist) – licensed for amyotrophic lateral sclerosis
- Non-invasive ventilation for advanced cases of breathlessness

Congenital syphilis

Examine this patient's face

The patient has a saddle-shaped nose. Examination of the eyes shows an interstitial keratitis. The patient has Hutchinson's incisors (peg-shaped incisors which are widely spaced), frontal bossing and a prominent mandible. I would also like to check the legs for sabre tibia.

These features are consistent with congenital syphilis.

How is this infection acquired?

- *T. pallidum* crosses the placenta after the first trimester.
- It is transmitted vertically, usually by an untreated mother.

What is late congenital syphilis?

- This is when the child develops signs of syphilis after 2 years of age, as found in this patient.
- It is similar to tertiary syphilis.
- Early congenital syphilis presents in the first few months of life and is equivalent to secondary syphilis.

What other clinical signs are there of late congenital syphilis?

- Perforated palate or nasal septum
- Deafness secondary to CN VIII nerve pathology
- Rhagades – linear scars at the angle of the mouth
- Clutton's joints – knee effusions
- Optic atrophy
- Retinopathy

What are the treatment options?

Prevention

- Treat syphilis early if picked up in the mother while pregnant

Medical

- Treat child with antibiotics

CENTRAL NERVOUS SYSTEM

Spastic paraparesis

Examine this patient's lower limbs

There is diffuse muscle wasting. The patient has increased tone in both legs. Power is decreased to 3/5 in all muscle groups. Ankle and knee jerks are brisk bilaterally. There is ankle clonus and plantars are extensor. There is a patchy, non-specific lack of sensation to light touch.

I would like to complete my examination by checking for other sensory modalities (joint position sense, vibration sense, temperature sensation). I would also like to check the upper limbs and the cerebellar system.

These findings are consistent with spastic paraparesis. Further history and examination would be required to elicit an underlying cause.

What else would you be looking for on examination?

- General inspection, e.g. for cachexia (might suggest malignancy)
- Wasting of the small muscles of the hand would indicate cervical pathology, e.g. cervical spondylosis, MND (remember – MND does not have sensory signs)
- Cerebellar pathology indicates multiple sclerosis or Friedreich's ataxia – posterior column signs also occur in multiple sclerosis
- Loss of sacral sensation or defective anal sphincter tone – this would suggest that S2–4 are affected

What are the causes of a spastic paraparesis?

Congenital/birth trauma

- Friedreich's ataxia
- Cerebral palsy
- Hereditary spastic paraplegia

Inflammatory

- Multiple sclerosis
- Myelitis

Structural

- Spinal cord compression
- Traumatic
- Syringomyelia

Infective

- HIV
- HTLV-1, tropical spastic paraplegia
- General paralysis of the insane (syphilis)
- Taboparesis (syphilis)

Vascular

- Anterior spinal artery thrombosis
- Atherosclerotic disease of spinal arteries
- Vasculitis e.g. PAN
- Arteriovenous malformation

Other causes

- MND
- Parasaggital meningioma
- Metastases
- Subacute combined degeneration of the cord

What are the causes of spinal cord compression?

- Spinal cord compression is a medical emergency.
- Look out for bladder/bowel involvement.

Causes

- Disc prolapse at L1/L2 or higher
- Epidural abscess
- Neoplastic – Hodgkin's lymphoma, myeloma, lung, breast, prostate, renal, thyroid
- Infective – spinal TB, epidural abscess
- Traumatic – fracture
- Paget's disease

How do you determine the site of the spinal lesion in a cord compression?

- Check for sensory level (this patient has normal sensation but it may apply to other patients)
- Examine sensation in different dermatomes
- When signs confined only to the lower limbs, then it is a T2/L1 lesion
- Loss of sphincter sensation and tone implies an S2–4 lesion

What investigations would you perform in this patient?

The overall clinical picture would guide me but in general I would carry out the following tests.

Bloods

- LFT
- Bone profile
- PSA (signs of metastases)
- FBC (anaemia)
- ESR (inflammatory/infective causes)
- Syphilis serology
- Vitamin B_{12} levels (SACD)
- HIV testing

Non-invasive tests

- CT of brain (space-occupying lesion)
- MRI of spinal cord (for plaques, syrinx, space-occupying lesion)

Invasive tests

- CSF (oligoclonal bands)

How might you distinguish clinically between a parasaggital meningioma and a thoracic cord compression?

- These two conditions can be difficult to distinguish on clinical examination.

- Both present with a spastic paraparesis, possible bladder involvement and sparing of upper limbs and possibly affect joint position sense.
- Parasaggital meningioma may cause focal neurological signs, seizures and headaches, as well as cortical sensory impairment in the lower limbs.
- Thoracic cord compression may present with back pain and a sensory level.

Cauda equina syndrome

Examine this patient's legs

The patient has a bilateral flaccid paralysis of the lower limbs with reduced tone and power. Knee and ankle jerks are absent. Sensation is decreased to light touch and this involves the saddle and perineal areas. I would like to check for anal sphincter tone.

The patient has signs of cauda equina syndrome.

What are the causes of this?

- Disc prolapse
- Metastases
- Cauda equina tumours. e.g. neurofibroma
- Epidural abscess

What other signs may this patient present with?

- Bladder symptoms – reduced bladder sensation (to filling and urethral sensation), incomplete emptying
- Painless urinary retention
- Faecal soiling

Why has this presented with lower motor neuron signs?

- The spinal cord ends at L1.
- Below this level, the peripheral nerve roots lie within the cauda equina. Any lesion here would cause LMN signs.

What investigation would you perform in such a patient?

- Urgent MRI

How would this be treated?

- Urgent surgical decompression

Cervical myelopathy

What is cervical myelopathy?

- In cervical myelopathy there is central cervical disc protrusion. This causes spinal cord compression. It will often occur at C4/5, C5/6 or C6/7 levels.
- The patient may be asymptomatic or complain of neck pain and/or difficulty in walking.

What would you expect to find on examination in a patient with this condition?

- Spastic paraparesis in the lower limbs ± involvement of spinothalamic tracts
- Inversion of biceps and supinator reflexes (absent jerks with brisk finger flexion suggesting that the defect is at C5/6 level)
- Small muscle wasting of hands – indicates C8/T1 lesion (uncommon)

What conditions cause cervical myelopathy?

- Cervical spondylosis (commonest cause)
- Spinal cord tumour
- Traumatic
- Osteoarthritis
- Ischaemia
- Congenital narrowing of spinal cord

What is the differential diagnosis for cervical myelopathy?

- Multiple sclerosis
- MND
- Syringomyelia
- Spinal cord tumour
- SACD

Which group of patients most commonly have cervical myelopathy?

- The elderly

What factors are thought to be responsible for cervical spondylosis?

- Degenerative changes
- Congenital narrowing of the spinal canal
- Ischaemic changes

What symptoms might the patient complain of?

- The signs in this condition are usually more pronounced than the symptoms
- Difficulty walking
- Neck pain (infrequent complaint)
- Weak or clumsy hands

What is the main investigation you would carry out in such a patient?

- MRI of the spine

What are the treatment options?

Conservative

- Monitoring
- Simple aids, e.g. collar or neck brace, cervical traction
- Analgesia for pain

Surgery

Decompression of the spinal cord by:

- cervical laminectomy *or*
- anterior fusion of vertebral bodies and disc removal.

Brown–Sequard syndrome

Examine this patient's neurological system in the lower limbs

The patient has upper motor neuron signs affecting only the left side. On the left side there is increased tone, decreased power to 3/5 in all muscle groups, brisk knee and ankle reflexes and extensor plantars.

Joint position sense and vibration are also compromised on the left side. Vibration sense is decreased up to the iliac crest. Pin-prick sensation is affected on the right side up to the umbilical region. At the umbilical region, there is a narrow zone of hyperaesthesia.

The patient has pyramidal signs and dorsal column signs on the left side and spinothalamic signs on the contralateral side.

I would like to check for bladder and bowel involvement. I would also like to confirm that temperature sensation is also affected on the right side.

The patient has Brown–Sequard syndrome at the T10 level.

Tell me about the defect in this condition

- This condition results from lateral hemisection of the spinal cord.
- This affects the dorsal columns, corticospinal tract and spinothalamic tracts on one side.
- Because the spinothalamic tracts cross over as they leave the spinal cord, pain and temperature sensations are affected contralaterally.

What are the causes of Brown–Sequard syndrome?

- Trauma, e.g. bullet and stab wounds
- Tumour
- Myeloma
- Infective – TB
- Multiple sclerosis
- Syringomyelia
- Vascular event

What would be the most important investigation to carry out?

- MRI scan of the spine

Absent ankle jerks and extensor plantars

Examine this patient's reflexes in the lower limbs

Tone and power are normal in the lower limbs. Sensation is intact. Examination of reflexes reveals extensor plantars and absent knee and ankle jerks.

I would like to examine the rest of the neurological system as well as dipstick the urine for glucose.

What are the possible causes for your findings?

- Diabetes
- Taboparesis
- MND
- Mixed cervical and lumbar pathology
- SACD
- Congenital causes, e.g. Friedreich's ataxia

What investigations would you carry out in this patient?

- Bloods – blood glucose, vitamin B_{12} level, syphilis serology
- Be guided by clinical signs but consider also:
  - muscle biopsy (MND)
  - MRI spinal cord (cervical/lumbar pathology).

Cerebellopontine angle lesions

Examine this patient's cranial nerves

There is decreased light touch sensation and power on the right side of the face (with sparing of the temporalis muscle, indicating an upper motor neuron lesion).

Hearing is also decreased on the right side with a normal Rinne's test. Weber's test lateralizes to the left ear. These signs indicate a sensorineural deficit in the right ear.

I would like to complete my examination by assessing the corneal reflex and the cerebellar system (for ipsilateral signs).

This patient has impairment of CNs V, VII and VIII on the right side, probably due to a cerebellopontine angle (CPA) lesion on the right side.

What is the most likely cause for this?

- Acoustic neuroma (vestibular schwannoma)

Name some other causes of a CPA lesion

Neoplastic

- Meningioma
- Astrocytoma of cerebellum
- Medulloblastoma of cerebellum
- Epidermoid tumours
- Pontine glioma
- Nasopharyngeal carcinoma
- Metastatic infiltration

Infective

- TB
- Syphilis

What other signs may this patient develop?

- CNs IX and X palsies
- Ipsilateral cerebellar signs
- Papilloedema (due to raised intracranial pressure)

Where is the CPA located?

- It is between the cerebellum and pons and is bordered by the petrous temporal bone.
- It is housed in a triangular fossa.

What investigations would you carry out in this patient?

Simple tests

- Syphilis serology
- Mantoux/Heaf testing if TB is suspected

Radiological tests

- Skull radiograph – may show enlargement of the internal auditory meatus
- CXR if TB is suspected
- MRI – demonstrates a space-occupying lesion
- CT scanning – may not detect smaller tumours, e.g. gliomas
- Angiography – helps identify vascular tumours, e.g. meningioma

Other

- Caloric testing – assessment of labyrinth function
- Audiometric testing – evidence of sensorineural hearing loss
- CSF testing – limited use

How would you treat acoustic neuroma?

- Arrange early neurosurgical assessment
- Conservative – monitoring with regular MRI scans for smaller tumours
- Radiotherapy
- Surgery – resection of tumour

Syringomyelia

Examine the neurological system in this patient's upper limbs

On general inspection this patient has a kyphosis. There is small muscle wasting in both hands and forearm. There are also numerous scars on both hands. The patient has Charcot's joints of the elbows. Tone is decreased in the arms. There is weakness in all muscle groups. Reflexes are absent bilaterally in the upper limbs. There is a dissociated sensory loss in both arms extending into the chest wall in a so-called 'cape distribution'.

This patient has signs consistent with syringomeyelia.

What do you mean by dissociated sensory loss?

- This refers to the fact that pain and temperature sensation are impaired but joint position sense, pain and light touch remain intact.

What else would you like to examine in this patient?

- Cerebellar system (due to involvement of the medial longitudinal bundle above C5)
- Face for dissociated sensory impairment (due to the syrinx affecting CN V)
- Eyes for Horner's syndrome (due to involvement of the sympathetic chain at C8/T1)
- Bulbar involvement (with a wasted tongue, palatal weakness, dysphagia, dysarthria)
- The lower limbs (for spastic paraparesis)
- Hands for la main succulente (cyanosed, cold, unsightly hands due to vasomotor impairment)
- Chest wall for dissociated sensation

Why do you think this patient has scars on his hands?

- Due to painless cuts and burns as a result of impaired pain and temperature sensation

What is a syrinx and what part of the spinal cord does it tend to affect?

- This is a fluid-filled slit like cavity either involving the spinal cord (myelia) or brainstem (bulbia). This cavity contains CSF.
- It is usually localized to one area of the spinal cord (usually the cervical region) but can extend to involve the whole spinal cord. The cause of this condition is unknown but is thought to be associated with alteration in CSF flow.
- The syrinx affects the anterior horn cells and spinothalamic tracts and eventually the corticospinal tracts. The dorsal columns are affected late on in the disease.

What might this condition be associated with?

- Arnold–Chiari malformation
- Hydrocephalus
- Spina bifida
- Congenital deformities at the foreman magnum

What would be the other differentials to consider in this patient?

- Cervical spondylosis
- Spinal cord pathology:
  - spinal cord tumours
  - spinal cord metastases
  - spinal cord haemorrhage/infarction
  - spinal cord trauma
- Neural tube defects
- Guillain–Barré syndrome

What investigations would you carry out in this patient?

Plain radiographs

- May show widened cervical canal and pick up craniovertebral deformity

CT myelography

- Myelogram shows up expanded cord around the syrinx
- Delayed high resolution CT scanning following myelography shows the syrinx filled with contrast medium

MRI

- **Investigation of choice**, will show up the syrinx with gadolinium-enhanced images

How would you manage this condition?

Supportive

- Neurorehabilitation and patient education

Medical

- There are no medical treatments yet available for this condition

Surgical

- Surgery produces mixed results. Options include:
  - suboccipital craniectomy and cervical laminectomy to relieve CSF pressure
  - drainage of the syrinx into the subarachnoid space
  - shunting: ventriculoperitoneal, lumboperitoneal or syringoperotoneal shunt
  - neuroendoscopic surgery – useful when there are multiple syrinxes

Dysarthria

- Dysarthria occurs when pronunciation is unclear but there is normal content and meaning to the speech.

Case 1

The patient has dysarthria with slurred/staccato speech. There are no features of expressive or receptive dysphasia. I would like to examine the cerebellar system and take a history.

The speech indicates cerebellar pathology.

Case 2

The patient has a dysarthric speech, which is monotonous and has little variation. The speech is slurred. I also note the expressionless face and fine resting tremor in the right hand.

I would like to perform a glabellar tap and examine the arms for cogwheeling/lead pipe rigidity. I would also expect to find a shuffling/festinating gait when the patient walks.

This patient has signs of Parkinsonism.

Case 3

This patient has a slurred, 'Donald Duck-like' speech. There is absent palatal movement and the patient cannot move the tongue forwards.

This patient has a pseudobulbar palsy, most likely due to infarct of both internal capsules.

How would you classify dysarthrias?

Ataxic

- Cerebellar disease

Spastic

- Parkinsonian
- Pseudobulbar palsy

Flaccid

- Bulbar palsy
- CVA

Mixed

- Brain trauma
- MND (amyotrophic lateral sclerosis)
- Multiple CVAs

Local problems

- Mouth ulcers
- Temporomandibular pathology

Cerebellar disease

Examine this patient's cerebellar system

The patient has a staccato, slurred speech. There is dysdiadochokinesia of the right hand with a right-sided intention tremor and past pointing. There is heel–shin ataxia at the right leg. The patient has horizontal nystagmus, which has its fast phase on the right-hand lateral gaze. Tone and reflexes in the right upper and lower limbs are decreased.

Examining the gait, the patient is unsteady and is falling towards the right-hand side. When the patient is asked to stand with his eyes closed, he leans towards the right-hand side. There is also rebound phenomenon.

The patient has cerebellar syndrome affecting the right-hand side.

What do you mean by rebound phenomena?

- This occurs when the patient is asked to hold his arms out in front.
- When moving the affected arm down, it recoils back past the starting point without control.

How might the patient present if the lesion was at the vermis?

- This would lead to bilateral signs.
- Truncal ataxia causes difficulty in sitting and standing. The patient has a waddling, wide-based gait, falling to both sides.

What are the underlying causes for this?

Commoner causes

- Alcohol
- Multiple sclerosis
- Brainstem infarct

Vascular

- Cerebellar haemorrhage/infarct
- Arteriovenous malformation

Infective

- HIV
- TB
- Abscess

Neoplastic

- Malignancy – primary or secondary
- Posterior fossa tumour, e.g. CPA tumours
- Paraneoplastic syndrome (usually from bronchial carcinoma)

Endocrine/metabolic

- Hypothyroidism

Toxic/therapeutic

- Phenytoin
- Lead poisoning
- Carbon monoxide exposure
- Solvent abuse

Congenital

- Hereditary ataxias, e.g. Friedreich's ataxia
- Congenital malformations, e.g. Arnold–Chiari malformation

What investigations would you perform in this patient?

Bloods

- TFTs (hypothyroidism)
- FBC, LFTs, GGT (signs of metastases/alcohol)
- Consider HIV testing and investigation for TB

Radiology

- CXR (signs of associated bronchial cancer)
- MRI scan (tumour/infarct, may also show up atrophic changes)

Other

- ECG
- Echocardiography
- Carotid Doppler studies (part of a vascular work-up)

How would you manage this patient?

- This is determined by the underlying cause, e.g. multiple sclerosis, chronic alcohol use.

Facial nerve palsy

Examine this patient's face

There is a left-sided facial weakness. This is evidenced by loss of the left nasolabial fold and drooping of the left side of the mouth. There is asymmetry when asking the patient to smile and blow out the cheeks. The patient is unable to raise the left eyebrow or to resist attempts to open the left eye when asked to keep it closed.

The patient has a lower motor neuron deficit affecting the left side.

Why is this a lower motor neuron deficit?

- Lower motor neuron lesions cause complete ipsilateral facial weakness.
- In upper motor neuron lesions, the forehead muscles are spared.

What else would you like to look for on examination?

- Examine the external auditory meatus – signs of herpes zoster and otitis media
- Examine the hearing – hyperacusis suggests involvement of the nerve to stapedius (within the petrous temporal bone)
- Examine taste sensation – loss in the anterior two-thirds suggests that the chorda tympani is involved (also within the petrous temporal bone)
- Corneal ulceration – due to defect in eye closure
- Parotid gland – signs of enlargement (which may compress the facial nerve)

What are the possible causes for this condition?

Common causes

- Bell's palsy
- Ramsay Hunt syndrome (due to herpes zoster)

Infective/inflammatory

- Multiple sclerosis
- Mumps parotitis
- Polio
- Otitis media
- Mononeuritis multiplex (see p. 129)

Vascular

- Pontine infarct
- Parotid tumour

Traumatic

- Skull fracture

Neoplastic

- CPA angle tumours

Name some causes of a bilateral lower motor neuron VII palsy

- Guillain–Barré syndrome
- Myasthenia gravis
- Other myopathic disorders, e.g. myotonic dystrophy
- Lyme disease
- Sarcoidosis

How would you diagnose Bell's palsy?

- This is a diagnosis of exclusion.
- Usually other causes can be reasonably excluded on clinical examination.
- If there is doubt then consider the following tests:

Bloods

- FBC, ESR
- Titres for CMV, herpes simplex virus (HSV), varicella zoster virus, hepatitis

Radiology

- Radiograph if fracture suspected
- MRI for suspected tumour

What do you know about Bell's palsy?

- Bell's palsy is an idiopathic condition.
- It is thought that it is related to a virus (possibly the herpes virus) that triggers an immune response damaging the facial nerve.

What is the prognosis for patients with Bell's palsy?

- The prognosis is usually very good, especially when there is partial Bell's palsy.
- Most patients recover spontaneously within 3–6 months (if partial Bell's, then usually with 2 weeks).
- 5% of patients have residual ophthalmic complications, e.g. dry eyes and corneal ulceration, and about the same proportion are left with long-term facial weakness.

How would you treat Bell's palsy?

Medical

This is controversial but the generally accepted treatments are:

- Steroids are most effective if started with 72 hours of onset.
- There is mixed evidence for use of aciclovir, but many advocate a 5-day course, again most effective if started within 72 hours of onset.

Ophthalmic complications

- Artificial tears in the day and lubricants at night
- Consider eye patch or shield
- Ophthalmology input for severe cases or if infection develops

Physiotherapy

- Useful for cases that are slow to recover

Hemiplegia

Examine this patient's peripheral nervous system

This elderly patient has a left-sided weakness in a pyramidal distribution. The left upper limb is held into the chest wall, with the elbow, wrist and fingers in flexion. In the left lower limb, the hip and knee are held in extension and the ankle is in plantar flexion. The left upper and lower limb have increased tone in all muscle groups and all reflexes are brisk. Plantars on the left side are extensor. There is decreased sensation to light touch in the left upper and lower limbs.

I note the presence of a facial muscle weakness on the left side. I would like to confirm that this is an upper motor neuron weakness (by confirming sparing of frontalis and orbicularis oculi) and check for a homonymous hemianopia and for signs of dysphasia and dysarthria. I would also like to examine the cardiovascular system.

The patient has hemiplegia affecting the left side, most likely caused by a stroke.

What other causes are there for hemiplegia?

CVA

- Thromboembolic – 80% of CVAs
- Intracerebral haemorrhage – 15% of CVAs

Other vascular

- Subarachnoid haemorrhage
- Subdural haematoma

Neoplastic

- Brain tumour

Infective

- Syphilis
- HIV

Inflammatory

- Autoimmune disease, e.g. antiphospholipid syndrome

Other

- Polycythaemia
- Trauma

What investigations would you carry out if presenting for the first time?

Bloods

- FBC
- ESR

- CRP
- FBG
- WCC
- Syphilis serology

Other

- ECG (looking for AF, recent MI)
- Carotid Doppler studies (for carotid atheroma)
- Echocardiography (for ventricular thrombus post MI, endocarditis)

Radiology

- CXR (identifies neoplasms)
- CT scanning – identifies infarct after 48 hours but can pick up haemorrhagic cause if done straight away
- Consider MRI (if suspecting a tumour or multiple sclerosis)

What drug treatments are useful in acute stroke?

Thromboembolic stroke

- Provided there are no contraindications, the evidence supports the use of thrombolysis (with intravenous alteplase) in a specialist stroke unit following immediate CT or MRI scanning (to exclude haemorrhagic stroke). Thrombolysis is more effective the sooner it is administered and up to 4.5 hours after an acute stroke. There must be a careful consideration of comorbidities as there is a risk of haemorrhage.
- If thrombolysis is not administered, then aspirin 300 mg should be given as quickly as possible once the diagnosis is made.

Haemorrhagic stroke

- No drug therapies available
- Some trials have found benefit from the use of administering haemostatic treatment (recombinant activated factor VIIa)

Multiple sclerosis (MS)

Examine this patient's legs

The patient has a spastic paraparesis of the lower limbs. There is also heel–shin ataxia. This suggests a cerebellar disorder, but I would like to conduct a full cerebellar and neurological examination.

These features are consistent with a demyelinating disease such as multiple sclerosis.

How would you define multiple sclerosis?

- MS is a chronic demyelinating condition affecting the brain and spinal cord. It is characterized by plaque formation which varies in both time and place.

What other signs may you elicit from a full clinical assessment?

- Optic neuritis
- Internuclear opthalmoplegia
- Spastic paraparesis
- Dorsal column involvement
- Bladder and bowel disturbances
- Sexual disturbances – impotence and ejaculatory failure
- Cerebellar signs
- Facial palsies
- Vertigo
- Mood disturbances
- Dementia
- Seizures

What are the different patterns of presentation for multiple sclerosis?

- Relapsing–remitting: most common variety (this is defined as a minimum of two acute flare-ups in the last 3 years, each followed by remission)
- Primary progressive
- Secondary progressive
- Progressive relapsing

What investigations would you carry out in this patient?

- Often rely on the history of a relapsing–remitting course
- MRI is the **investigation of choice** – will usually show up plaques and characteristic lesions in brain and spinal cord
- CSF – oligoclonal bands and raised white cells
- Visual or auditory evoked potentials show prolonged latency if demyelination is present

What are the management options for such patients?

Supportive

- Physiotherapy and occupational therapy input
- Patient education and advice on support groups
- Neurology follow-up, including specialist neurological rehabilitation
- Dietary measures – increased intake of linoleic acid (found in corn, soya and sunflower)
- Influenza vaccination

Medical

- Treat acute flare-ups with steroids.
- Treat complications, e.g.
  - urinary incontinence – anticholinergics (e.g. oxybutinin)
    – intermittent self-catheterization, intravesical
    – botulinum toxin in certain cases

- impotence in men – sildenafil
- spasticity – baclofen and gabapentin
- pressure sores prevention

- Interferon-β is licensed for relapsing–remitting and secondary progressive multiple sclerosis. The evidence supports reduced relapse rates in some cases.
- Glatiramer for relapsing–remitting multiple sclerosis, especially in those patients that are mobile.
- Other options include intravenous immunoglobulin, plasma exchange and azathioprine.

I STATION 4 COMMUNICATION SKILLS AND ETHICS

Case 1

Information for the candidate

You are the junior doctor in A&E. Mrs Jones is a 35-year-old secretary who presented with a 2-day history of headache and vomiting. On examination you find she has neck stiffness, photophobia and fever. Bloods show a neutrophilia with an elevated CRP. CT scan of the brain is normal. You wish to rule out meningitis and therefore need to consent her for a lumbar puncture (LP). She is a widow and lives with her 5-year-old daughter who is well.

Please discuss the findings so far and obtain her consent for an LP.

Brief for the actor

You are a 35-year-old woman who until now has been fit and well. For the past 2 days you have suffered a gradually worsening headache, which is now severe. Today you have vomited several times and are now quite feverish and your neck is stiff. You have a 5-year-old daughter who is your main concern. Your husband died tragically 2 years ago in a car crash, and there are no other relatives in this country. You are now in the hospital having just had some blood tests and a brain scan. The doctor is about to come and speak to you. You are anxious to know what is wrong, but your main concern is the safety and welfare of your daughter. You start off the conversation by wanting to self-discharge or to take antibiotics at home. You do not want to leave your daughter with anyone. If gently persuaded, you will reluctantly agree to have the LP, provided your neighbour (whom you get on well with) agrees to look after your daughter. However, you want to be assured this has been very carefully arranged before you agree.

Preparation

Make sure that you appreciate the main points in the history

- Provisional diagnosis of meningitis
- Requires informed consent for LP
- Social set-up, i.e. seems to be sole carer for her daughter

Ethical issues

- Informed consent – capacity to consent and details specific to procedure
- Welfare and safety of child while mother is being treated

Discussion with the patient

Introduction

- Introduce yourself and state the purpose of the consultation.
- Show empathy, enquire how she is feeling.

Explanation of provisional diagnosis

- Explain the results of tests done so far, i.e. bloods and CT of brain.
- Discuss why you need to exclude meningitis as a cause for her symptoms.
- Early on, check her understanding of meningitis and respond to any questions.
- Explain how meningitis is diagnosed (LP) and managed.
- Explain the importance of identifying meningitis to aid tracing and treatment of contacts, including her daughter.

Consent for LP

- Check her capacity to consent. Check she is not confused and is able to provide informed consent.
- Discuss why the procedure is being proposed and what it means in terms of management, i.e. admission to hospital and IV antibiotics for several days.
- Explain what the procedure entails in a step-wise logical manner using appropriate lay terminology.
- Explain post-procedure care, e.g. she will need to lie down flat for 4–6 hours.
- Identify any contraindications, such as coagulopathies, allergies or relevant medication, such as warfarin.
- Discuss any alternative strategies, such as treating empirically with first-line antibiotics and monitoring for response, but emphasize this is not ideal.
- Discuss the consequences of not carrying out a lumbar puncture, e.g. uncertain diagnosis, incorrect antibiotic usage.

Addressing the needs of the child

- An important consideration for the mother will be the care of her daughter while she is undergoing investigation and treatment, so it will be important to address this during your discussions.
- Emphasize that it is in her daughter's best interests for the patient to be fully treated.
- Enquire about her social set-up and any family, friends or neighbours who can help with her care.
- If there is no one available to care for her daughter while she is in hospital, you would need to speak to your seniors, the paediatricians and social services about providing temporary care.

Summarize the main points of your discussion and agree an action plan.

Discussion with the examiner

Potential areas of discussion include:

What will you do if the patient refuses a lumbar puncture?

- Negotiation is key and, if you can successfully address the patient's main concern, it is likely that you will persuade her to have the LP.
- It might also be useful to point out that carrying out a LP would also be in her daughter's best interest because it would help in determining treatment for contacts.

How can you be certain that she has capacity to provide consent?

You can consider someone as having capacity if he or she:

- Understands the information
- Retains the information
- Can adequately consider the risks and benefits of the proposed management plan (Mental Capacity Act 2005)
- Can communicate the information.

What are the main ethical considerations in this case?

- It is important to always respect the patient's autonomy, **provided that** she has the capacity to make this decision. She will need informed consent to best make up her mind. Aim for an outcome that benefits the patient medically in terms of managing her condition while at the same time addressing her main concerns regarding her daughter. The best outcome is one that achieves both of these objectives.
- Try to prevent an outcome that will do physical or emotional harm to the patient. This includes addressing the mother's concerns about her daughter.
- There may be conflict between these ethical principles, e.g. preserving someone's right to refuse life-saving treatment (autonomy) when they do not have the capacity to make their own decision (so balancing autonomy with beneficence). In this particular case, however, the patient has capacity so it is likely that treatment cannot be forced upon her.
- Informed consent should involve the purpose of the procedure and the potential alternatives, as well as any significant risks and benefits. It should also include the consequences of not performing the procedure and aspects of the procedure with aftercare details.

What options are there for care of the daughter?

- Discussed above under 'Discussion with the patient'.

How long might you allow this patient to decide on whether or not she will proceed with the LP?

The explanation about the procedure would include information about the nature of meningitis, how rapidly it can progress and the need to act urgently to carry out the LP so that treatment can be initiated. However, if the patient has capacity and says she needs time, then you would want to accommodate her while at the same time emphasizing the risks of delays.

Are there any circumstances under which you would consider performing the LP without her consent?

- If she was confused owing to the meningitis and demonstrated that she does not have capacity.
- If she arrested before she had the chance to provide informed consent.

Other similar cases that might involve 'consent'

- Consent for an emergency operation, e.g. coronary angiography
- Consent from a relative for an incapacitated patient, e.g. DNR (do not resuscitate) status
- Consent from a patient who lacks capacity
- Consent for advanced care planning, such as refusing treatment

Case 2

Information for the candidate

You are the junior doctor on call. A crash call was put out for Mr Smith, which you attended along with your team. Attempts to resuscitate him proved unsuccessful and were stopped after 30 minutes. Mr Smith was an 83-year-old man, admitted 10 days ago with right lower lobe pneumonia. His medical history consists of well-controlled hypertension. He had been under the care of the geriatric team, who are not around as it is late in the day, and you are part of the on-call team. Nursing staff report that at the consultant ward round today Mr Smith and his wife were told that he had made a good recovery and would be discharged tomorrow. Having looked through the notes you are satisfied the relevant test results and examination findings had improved and this had been well documented.

This evening Mr Smith complained of mild chest pain shortly before losing consciousness.

You are now asked to explain to Mrs Smith what has happened and address the fact that she had been told earlier that everything was okay.

Brief for the actor

You are a 79-year-old woman called Mrs Smith. Your husband was admitted to hospital with a bad chest infection 10 days ago, and earlier today his consultant was very pleased with his recovery. Discharge had been set for tomorrow morning. This evening as you were coming back to the ward you saw a number of doctors running into your husband's room. You were asked to wait in the patient waiting room. When given the news that your husband is dead it will come as a shock. You will not understand why you were told earlier that all was well and how this has happened.

You will also want to know exactly what has happened between the earlier ward round and now.

Preparation

Make sure that you appreciate the main points

- Breaking bad news about the death
- The need to explain to the wife why this patient was declared fit for discharge and yet died suddenly later that day
- Recognize and deal professionally with the fact that you are not this patient's regular doctor but taking responsibility as the doctor on call

Ethical and communication issues

- It is vital to show sensitivity and compassion throughout the case.
- As part of probity it is important to be open and honest about the events that took place.
- Be prepared to say you do not know something and be willing to find out and liaise with Mr Smith's regular team when it is back on duty.

Discussion with the patient's wife

Introduction

- Introduce yourself and clarify whom you are speaking to and that she is related to the patient.
- Consider the setting – best to be seated in a private room, with tissues handy and a nurse present, and ask if there is anyone else she would like with her.
- Ask Mrs Smith what she already knows – she may already suspect.

Explanation of events

- Fire a warning shot e.g. '… I have some bad news for you.'
- Explain the events that took place today, e.g. 'Mr Smith has been treated for a chest infection, which has responded well to treatment, and I gather today he was well enough for discharge. However, this evening, he became suddenly unwell and complained of chest pain. Unfortunately, his heart stopped beating and, although we did everything we could to bring him back, we were not successful. I am very sorry to have to tell you that your husband has passed away.'
- Allow for pauses and be guided by Mrs Smith's reaction.
- Enquire how she is feeling.
- Address why Mr Smith might have suddenly deteriorated. If necessary, go through the series of events from when Mr Smith was admitted to hospital until now. Back up what you say by referring in simple terms to the investigation/ examination results.
- Be honest, and say when you do not know the answers and offer to come back to her on these. Explain likely possibilities, such as unexpected heart attack or pulmonary embolism. Be prepared to explain what these are in lay terms.

Address what happens next

- Offer a chance for Mrs Smith to speak to the regular team when back on duty and offer to facilitate this meeting.
- Explain that one of the doctors will speak to the coroner and take advice on whether a post mortem is indicated. This needs to be decided before certification of the death can take place.
- Take the wife's views on post mortem (this suggestion may upset her) and enquire about any special considerations with regard to the funeral, e.g. Jewish funerals need to be within 24 hours of death.

Agree an action plan before leaving

- Discuss whether she would like to see her husband, or speak with the regular team in the morning.
- Ensure that a nurse or relative is with her before leaving. Offer to arrange for her to see the hospital chaplain.
- Offer to speak to her again later if she wishes.

Discussion with the examiner

Potential areas of discussion include:

What are your views about performing a post mortem on Mr Smith?

- This patient's death occurred suddenly and unexpectedly and while he was in hospital. For these reasons, the case should be discussed with the coroner, who will decide on a post mortem.
- The advantages of a post mortem are that it would provide a cause of death, which might help the family understand better what has happened. It may also help the clinical team with their training and hopefully prevent a similar problem occurring again.
- The family may not feel comfortable with a full examination, in which case a limited examination could be carried out.

In general, why might you report a death to the coroner?

- Suspicious circumstances, e.g. violence, poisoning or neglect
- Accidental cause
- Resulting from hospitalization or from medical treatment
- Sudden or unexpected death
- Where the deceased had not been seen by a doctor within the past 14 days

What causes of sudden death are possible in this patient?

- Acute MI
- PE
- Dissecting aortic aneurysm
- Fatal cardiac arrhythmia
- Intracerebral haemorrhage (would not explain the chest pain)

What processes should be carried out following this incident? By this, I mean significant event analysis.

- Looking at the series of events leading up to the death in detail and making necessary changes to decrease the chances of this happening again

To what extent are you responsible for this patient and his relatives, given that you are not part of the regular team?

- Regardless of not being part of the regular team, there is an ethical and moral duty to provide the patient with the best possible care. Part of this involves dealing with relatives, especially when it comes to breaking bad news about death, however difficult this may be.
- In this regard while on call your team and you are responsible for any complications or problems occurring among medical patients.

Variations on the theme of 'breaking bad news'

- Telling someone that he or she has terminal cancer
- Telling someone that he or she has a chronic disease, e.g. epilepsy, inflammatory bowel disease, Huntington's chorea

Tips

This is a particularly challenging consultation as there is a lot to cover in the 14 minutes, and it will vary according to what bad news you are imparting. In addition, you need to deal with the deceased patient's wife in a calm, patient and professional manner.

Case 3

Information for the candidate

Mr Roberts is a 35-year-old man who was admitted 5 days ago following a road traffic accident. He sustained a significant head injury and was admitted to the intensive care unit (ICU). A CT scan revealed a subdural haematoma with significant midline shift. He was taken off sedation yesterday and is now on artificial ventilation. He is haemodynamically stable. The neurosurgeons, physicians and ICU consultant agree that the prognosis is extremely poor. Two doctors have certified him brainstem dead.

Please speak to his wife about the diagnosis and seek permission for organ donation.

Brief for the actor

You are a 32-year-old woman whose husband was involved in a car crash 5 days ago. The news came through to you at work. You dropped everything and have been at the hospital most of the time since. You are tired and have hardly slept over the past 5 days. John, your husband, has been in a coma ever since the crash and has been on a life support machine. You have been married 3 years and have a 1-year-old baby boy, who is currently with your parents who live locally. John and you never discussed the possibility of becoming incapacitated. If asked, John did not carry a donor card and you do not know what his view would have been on organ donation. You know deep down inside that John was a very giving person and that he probably would have wanted his organs donated (although you do not have to disclose this). Removing his organs is something that would make you feel very uncomfortable. Nursing staff have suggested that the outlook for John seems very bad, but you are quite anxious to hear directly from one of the doctors. If your concerns and anxieties are addressed, you agree to consider organ donation but state that you will need time (to be negotiated, but 2–3 hours to liaise with other family).

Preparation

Make sure that you appreciate the main points

- Breaking bad news about brainstem death and that there is no possibility of recovery
- Seek consent for use of organs for transplantation

Ethical and communication issues

- Vital to show sensitivity and compassion throughout the case
- Consider Mr Roberts' wishes and balance these with those of his wife

Discussion with the patient's wife

Introduction

- Introduce yourself and clarify whom you are speaking to.
- Consider the setting – best to be seated in a private room, with tissues handy and a nurse present, and ask if there is anyone else she would like present.
- Ask Mrs Roberts what she already knows – she may already suspect.

Explanation of events

- Fire a warning shot, e.g. '… I have some bad news for you.'
- Explain the events that have taken place, e.g. 'Mr Roberts was admitted with a significant head injury from which he has not regained consciousness in spite of all our efforts. Today we have carried out brainstem tests to assess whether he is likely to recover.'
- Explain what brainstem death is and that the diagnosis was made by two doctors – emphasize that Mr Roberts is being kept alive artificially and there is no chance of recovery. Remember that, according to the legal definition, Mr Roberts is already dead.
- Explain that the ventilation will be kept going until relatives have a chance to say goodbye.

Request for organ donation

- Enquire whether Mr Roberts had expressed any wishes regarding organ donation or if he carried an organ donation card.

- Discovering what Mr Roberts' wishes are may not be easy, especially if he has not stated his wishes or did not carry a donor card. This is where effective communication skills are important, because it would be your job to try to elucidate this information from his wife.
- Enquire how she and the rest of the family would feel about organ donation – obviously he cannot be brought back, but his organs could prolong someone else's life.
- Consider the fact that the patient and/or relatives may prefer certain organs being donated.
- Explain what will happen if organ donation is pursued, i.e. the transplant coordinator will be alerted and checks will be carried out to ensure that there are no contraindications and Mr Roberts will remain on ventilator support until the organs are removed.
- Allow her time to think about it and discuss it with the rest of her family and arrange a time to make a decision and take further questions.

Discussion with the examiner

How long would you allow Mrs Roberts to consider the issue about organ donation?

- There is no right or wrong answer here. Much will depend on the individual situation, including how the next of kin responds, denial about what has happened, religious objections to switching off the ventilator, etc.
- In the context of the scenario, the best way to approach this in the real life setting would be to negotiate with the next of kin and probably carry out the counselling in stages, i.e. come back later. This might help the next of kin come to terms with the situation better and liaise with other family members.

How long would you keep the patient on a ventilator?

- Once agreement is sought from the next of kin ventilation continues until the organs are removed.

How is brainstem death diagnosed?

- Criteria for diagnosis:
  - absent respiration with deep coma
  - absence of reversible causes, e.g. sedating drugs, hypoxia, electrolyte disturbances, hypoglycaemia, acidosis, hypothermia.
- Brainstem tests should be conducted by two appropriately qualified doctors 24 hours apart. The tests consist of:
  - fixed/dilated and unresponsive pupils
  - absent gag reflex
  - absent corneal reflex
  - absent vestibulo-ocular reflex
  - absent motor response in cranial nerves
  - lack of respiratory effort on removal of ventilator and rise in P_{CO_2} > 6.6 kPa

What is persistent vegetative state?

- This is a condition in which brainstem function is present in the absence of cortical control.
- Medically it is defined as a wakeful unconscious state. Legally it is not seen as death, which is where the controversy often arises.

What will be your response if Mrs Roberts refuses donation of her husband's organs?

Ultimately the organs belong to the patient, and it is his wishes that we would need to respect the most, i.e. his autonomy to decide if his organs are donated after death. However, if the family disagree, then this would put you in a difficult situation. You would want to maintain sensitivity at all times and would want to discuss it with your consultant and take further advice.

What would you do if the patient has a donor card and his wife refuses?

If the patient has a donor card or is on the organ donation register, then it is not legally necessary to have the family on board. However, in practice it is always best to seek agreement from the family, especially as this will be a very difficult time for them.

From a medical point of view, in which groups of patients would organ donation be unsuitable?

- Viral infections, e.g. HIV, hepatitis B and C, CJD
- Malignancy

Other similar cases

- Request from a live donor to donate to a relative, e.g. a patient with renal failure whose son wishes to donate a kidney.

Case 4

Information for the candidate

You are the junior doctor in the infectious disease clinic. Your next patient is Mr Balls, a 29-year-old gentleman with a 5-month history of TB. He has completed 4 months of triple therapy. Mr Balls has only recently moved into the local area. He was previously under a TB clinic at another hospital within the UK. Most of the medical records are in front of you but they do not confirm whether an HIV test was performed. Because Mr Balls is new to your clinic, you have performed a full clerking. You are about to clarify whether Mr Balls has had previous HIV testing.

Brief for the actor

You are a 29-year-old Caucasian gentleman. You are at the infectious disease department at the local hospital in London. You were diagnosed with TB after coughing blood and losing weight about 4-5 months ago, and have been on treatment since. You recently transferred to this new TB clinic after moving from Leeds where you were seeing a specialist there. You are concordant with your medications and were referred by your new GP to the local TB clinic to ensure you were being followed up. You worked as a security guard in Leeds but lost your job when the company went bankrupt. You moved to London with your wife because you found a job as a lorry driver. You have never used recreational drugs.

If asked, you recall being offered an HIV test and a full sexual health check at the TB clinic in Leeds. However, you declined the test because your wife was with you in the consultation. You have been married to Tracy for five years and both of you had a sexual health checkup up when you entered the relationship. Both of you tested negative for HIV and had no other STIs. To your knowledge, Tracy has been faithful. However, you had an affair for months that started about 1 year ago. You were sexually active with a female colleague at work called Sharon and often did not bother using a condom since she was on the contraceptive pill. You do not use condoms when having sex with your wife because she is also on the contraceptive pill. You have been willing to have the HIV test in the Leeds clinic but declined because you did not want your wife to know you had sex with another woman.

You are keen for your wife not to find out about your affair and want this information to be kept confidential. Your relationship with Sharon ended because she was cheating on you. Very recently she called you up. She was drunk and mentioned she was a sex worker a couple of years ago for a few months. As a result, you are worried about the possibility of having an STI but are still reluctant to have any tests because your affair might come to light. If the doctor suggests an HIV test, you will be reluctant to do this. However, you can be persuaded to change your mind provided the doctor is sympathetic to your concerns and answers your questions.

Preparation

Make sure you appreciate the main points

- Establish the need for an HIV test and offer pre-test counselling
- Appreciate any other risks factors for HIV or sexually transmitted infections in general
- Consider risks to any other sexual partners
- Explain the risk of Mr Balls having HIV

Ethical and communication issues

- Reassure Mr Balls that the information remains confidential but if he does have HIV then as part of contact tracing both Sharon and Tracy would have to be informed that they are at risk
- Remain non-judgemental throughout the consultation
- Enquire about any fears and concerns

Patient discussion

Introduction

- Introduce yourself and clarify whom you are speaking to
- Enquire about occupation
- Comment on the good news that the TB has been treated

Establishing understanding and risk factors

- Clarify whether Mr Balls was offered an HIV test at the previous clinic and what the outcome was.
- Ask about previous history and testing for HIV, hepatitis B and C and other STIs.
- Enquire about risk factors for HIV:
  - sexual partners including sexuality, ethnicity, contact with sex workers
  - recreational drugs
  - previous blood transfusions (particularly in developing countries)
- Enquire about any concerns regarding STIs.
- Ask what he knows about HIV and briefly explain in lay terms what it is, its natural history and mode of transmission.
- Emphasize there that there is a risk that Mr Balls has HIV.

Explain the reasons for being tested

- Put it to him that it is in his best interests to be tested.
- Comment on the benefits of being tested, explaining that if the test is negative it will offer peace of mind. If positive then early treatment and intervention can be offered, transmission of HIV infection to others can be prevented.
- Discuss the disadvantages of testing e.g. workplace discrimination, increased anxiety.
- Discuss the distinction between confidential testing and anonymous testing.
- Consider the option of not testing and the pros and cons of this.

HIV testing

- State that the test consists of a simple blood test.
- Offer to test for hepatitis B and C.
- Mention that there are many different types of HIV blood tests but most results are back within 24 hours.
- A negative test does not guarantee absence of HIV. You would then need to repeat the test in 3 months.

Implications of a positive test

- Reiterate that treatments are highly effective nowadays.
- Explain that if positive he would be referred to a specialist in HIV medicine.
- Discuss insurance applications: difficulty in taking out life insurance and getting a mortgage. However, taking the test and having a negative result should not affect his ability to get insurance.
- Address implications for employment.
- Explain that he would be unable to donate blood.
- A positive result does not mean he has AIDS. Explain the difference between HIV and AIDS.

- Emphasize that he can pass on the disease to other partners and must use precautions.
- He would need to pursue contact tracing if there are any exposed contacts.

Summarising and follow-up

- Offer opportunity to answer questions.
- Ask him if he wants the test. If he is unsure, then offer the opportunity to come back to you.
- If it becomes necessary, let him know that confidentiality can be broken if others are knowingly put at risk.
- Provide him with written material to take away.
- Tackle any other high-risk activities, particularly emphasising the importance of safe sex.
- Offer post-test counselling.

Discussion with examiner

Potential areas of discussion include:

Name some AIDS-defining conditions

- TB or any mycobacterial infection
- Kaposi's sarcoma
- CMV retinitis
- *Pneumocystis carinii* pneumonia
- Toxoplasmosis of the brain

If Mr Balls is found to have HIV, then how can you say you are keeping his information confidential if you are also saying that his partners would have to be told?

- Where possible confidentiality should always be withheld as this is important for the doctor–patient relationship.
- In this scenario an effort should be made firstly to explain the importance of informing the other sexual partners himself. If he is adamant you could ask him to think about it seriously and return in 1–2 days.
- If he remains unwilling to do this then you would have to let him know that you are allowed to break confidentiality owing to the risk of transmitting infection.

In which other instances could you break a patient's confidentiality?

- For notifiable diseases
- Where it is deemed in the public interest e.g. threat of murder/terrorism, driving against DVLA guidelines
- Due to a court order
- Acting in the patient's best interests e.g. if mental health issues or if in an unconscious state

Case 5

Information for the candidate

You are the FY2 doctor in the neurology clinic. Your next patient is Mr Bond, who is a fit and well 25-year-old man. He has been referred because his father has recently been diagnosed with Huntington's chorea. There is no other known family history of this disease. Mr Bond would like to be tested.

Please counsel him for this test.

Brief for the actor

You are a 25-year-old man. Your father was recently diagnosed as having Huntington's chorea following a few months' history of being very fidgety and agitated. There is no other history of any illnesses in the family. You have a brother aged 20 and a sister aged 17, neither of whom has been tested so far. You have asked your GP to refer you to be tested for the disease as you are worried about developing it. You have little knowledge about the condition and are not sure what could be offered if you have it. When asked if you want the test you will eventually decide against having it on the basis that there is no prevention or cure available, but you will want to consider the implications for future children and family.

Preparation

Make sure that you appreciate the main points in the history

- Establish the reasons for wanting the test.
- Discuss Huntington's chorea and its inheritance.
- Provide pre-test counselling.

Ethical issues

- Discussion about testing other family members
- Implications for future children

Discussion with the patient

Introduction

- Introduce yourself

Clarify the reason for the referral

- Enquire about the reason for referral.
- Ask about his father's recent diagnosis of Huntingdon's chorea, what complications he has had and how he is now, e.g. movement problems, dementia.
- Ask about his concerns and expectations.
- Enquire about known family members to compile a family tree and ask about any other known family history.

Check the patient's understanding

- Check his understanding of Huntington's, its risks and complications.
- Educate him on aspects he does not know about, including the natural history, treatment and prognosis of the condition.
- Explain the autosomal dominant pattern of inheritance of this condition and what this means for him. This should include his likely risk of having the condition (50%) and the risk to his children if he has the condition. If necessary draw out your explanation of the inheritance.
- Explain the idea behind genetic anticipation, i.e. that Huntington's chorea may present more severely and earlier in subsequent generations.

Implications of having Huntington's chorea

- For future children, i.e. 50% chance of passing it on and prenatal diagnosis as an option
- Medically
- Psychological impact
- Social impact, e.g. declaration to insurance companies, employment
- Discuss treatment options and emphasize that there is no cure
- Informing other family members that he has the condition and dealing with their anxieties/worries about the prospect of them having it if they are at risk or have not been tested

Explain the reasons for being tested

- If the test is negative, it will offer peace of mind. If it is positive, then early treatment and intervention can be offered and will identify the risk of transmitting the disease to future children. The test may also help with career planning.
- Discuss the disadvantages of testing, e.g. discrimination, increased anxiety, no prevention or cure available for the condition. There are also reports of patients developing 'survivor guilt' if they have a negative test. Also, a positive test will not predict the age of onset/severity of the condition.
- Consider the option of not testing and the pros and cons of this.

Information about the test

- A blood test would be used to analyse DNA (on the short arm of chromosome 4).
- There is the possibility of an incorrect test.
- Offer post-test counselling to go through the result.

Summarizing and follow-up

- Offer the opportunity to ask questions.
- Check if he wants the test. If he is unsure, then offer him the opportunity to come back to you or to come back with another family member.

- Ensure that the patient is not under any pressure from other individuals to take the test.
- Suggest that other family members are tested.
- Provide him with written material to take away.
- Arrange a meeting with a genetic counsellor.
- Enquire about siblings and suggest that they are tested.

Discussion with the examiner

Potential areas of discussion include:

Discuss what your strategies would be if the test result comes back positive

- It is important that formal post-test counselling be available with a genetic counsellor.
- It should be carried out according to the 'breaking bad news' case.

Why do you think that no other family members have been diagnosed with Huntington's chorea other than the father?

- Relatives may not have disclosed their diagnosis.
- Relatives may not have been tested for the condition.
- Relatives might not have developed the condition badly enough to present with it (which may reflect genetic anticipation).
- Relatives may have been lucky enough not to have inherited the condition.

What are the ethical considerations to think about if Mr Bond says to you that he wants the test but does not wish to share the result with anybody else?

- It is important to follow confidentiality but check his reasons for this request.
- Consider the issues of patient autonomy and avoiding psychological harm.
- Ensure that he has informed consent and understands the implications of withholding a positive result, i.e. from family, children.
- The other issue would be to check how you think he will deal emotionally with a positive result and whether lack of support might have a detrimental effect on him.

Variations on a theme of 'genetic counselling'

- Counselling a patient whose parent has been diagnosed with another inherited neurodegenerative condition, e.g. spinocerebellar ataxias (autosomal dominant, autosomal recessive and X-linked recessive types)
- Counselling a woman whose father has been diagnosed with adult-onset polycystic disease (autosomal dominant)

Case 6

Information for the candidate

You are the junior doctor in the endocrine clinic. The next patient is Mr Hoe. He is a 40-year-old man who has been a heavy goods vehicle driver for the past 17 years.

He has type II diabetes with no other significant past medical history. A month ago your consultant started him on insulin, as his diabetic control has remained poor despite oral medication, including metformin, sulfonylureas and sitagliptin. He has no retinopathy, but he has mild microalbuminuria and is hypertensive, taking ramipril. His HbA1c levels have been persistently raised above 10 for the past year. Today he has come to see you for a routine appointment. His feet and eyes were checked last month. You have received a letter from the GP mentioning that Mr Hoe is still driving. Of note, Mr Hoe is married with two young children and is the main breadwinner. His BP is 140/80 mmHg, urine dipstick negative, pulse 84 beats/minute, BMI 27 kg/m^2.

Please assess the patient's progress and address the issue of driving with him. You are not expected to take a full history.

Brief for the actor

You are a 40-year-old man and have worked as a heavy goods vehicle driver for most of your working life. You work for a large supplies company. You have had type II diabetes for 8 years and for most of that time were taking tablets. A month ago you were told that the diabetes was very badly controlled and that you required insulin treatment. You were reluctant in the first place, but your wife encouraged you to go ahead. The last month has been very difficult for you and the family. You tend to work very erratic hours and find it a chore to have to take your insulin on time, but your wife reminds you. In terms of administering the insulin, this has been fine. Your blood sugar control seems to have improved and you have expereinced no hypoglycaemic spells. Your wife stays at home to look after the children. The children are 7 and 4 years old. Now that you have started taking insulin, you have been advised that you need to stop driving but you need the income to support your family. You have until now ignored the advice and have not informed DVLA. You do not want to give up your job and do not see why you should have to take this advice. If presented with the reasons for having to give up driving, the implications of what will happen if you continue driving heavy goods vehicles and what the alternatives are, then you will accept the doctor's advice.

Preparation

Make sure that you appreciate the main points

- Enquire how he is managing with insulin, including compliance and complications.
- He holds a group 2 licence – according to the DVLA he cannot drive heavy goods vehicles while treated with insulin.
- There are significant social issues to address if he gives up his job.

Ethical and communication issues

- Aim to maintain the doctor–patient relationship by trying not to break confidentiality – for this reason you would need to encourage the patient to inform the DVLA himself and to give up driving heavy goods vehicles.
- If he is unwilling to stop driving, you would ultimately be legally and morally obligated to inform DVLA yourself in order to help protect the public (comes under the ethical principle of 'justice').

Discussion with the patient

Introduction

- Introduce yourself and clarify your role.

Enquiry about insulin

- Refer back to the last consultation and clarify what was decided.
- Clarify how he is getting on with insulin – compliance, blood sugars, ask about any hypoglycaemic episodes, problems relating to injecting/insulin pen.
- Enquire about his concerns and any queries about insulin.
- Clarify *briefly* his awareness of the reasons for treating diabetes.

General social enquiry

- Enquire further about his job and how taking insulin and having diabetes is affecting him on a daily basis.
- Ask about his wife and children, schooling, how he is managing financially and what other source of income there may be.

Addressing his driving

- Find out if he is aware of the DVLA regulations for group 2 licence drivers.
- If so, enquire about his reasons for continuing to drive.
- Encourage him to inform the DVLA and to stop driving. Explain the reason for the DVLA ruling, that it is to protect him and the public from a terrible accident if he has a hypoglycaemic episode at the wheel.
- Be guided according to how he reacts. If necessary, emphasize the implications of the impact on his wife and children if something were to happen.

Informing DVLA

- If Mr Hoe is not willing to stop driving, then keep trying to persuade him. Offer to speak to his wife and offer him a second opinion or the chance to speak to your consultant.
- You would need to explain to him that he is legally obliged to inform DVLA and that, if he does not, you would be duty bound to inform DVLA yourself.

Addressing his social needs

- Address any concerns and worries about having to stop driving.
- Focus particularly on his having to give up work and the knock-on effect of loss of income.
- Explore alternative options of taking other work, the possibility of transferring to group 1 licence driving, office/management work, etc. It may be best for him to negotiate with his boss if he is an employee. Offer to write a letter to his employer.
- Discuss the option of benefits, e.g. incapacity benefit, and discussion with a social worker. Also offer him they chance to speak to a counsellor.

Agree an action plan before he leaves

- Recognize that this is a big upheaval for this patient and accordingly maintain a sympathetic, supportive approach.
- Offer to speak to him and his wife if that will help. Arrange early follow-up.
- To successfully complete this case, the issue of driving and informing DVLA must be resolved. If necessary offer him a chance to speak to the consultant.

Discussion with the examiner

Potential areas of discussion include:

What would you say to Mr Hoe if he proposed to stop his insulin as a solution to the problem?

I would want to ensure that Mr Hoe is provided with informed consent for such an action. I would discuss the pros and cons of such action, as well as raise the possibility of alternatives to insulin. As he has tried metformin, sitagliptin and sulfonylureas, the main alternative would be a GLP-1 mimetic, e.g. exenatide, liraglutide. These are administered as twice-daily injections without the risk of hypoglycaemic episodes. However, this group of drugs is currently recommended for patients with a BMI > 35 kg/m^2 as they can cause weight loss.

It would be important to emphasize the reasons why insulin was started, i.e. because his diabetes was poorly controlled on oral medication, which would have been due to his pancreas having very little insulin of its own. Having high blood sugar would significantly increase his risk of macro- and microvascular complications and result in an increased tendency to infections. Insulin would help slow the progression of these complications and reduce the risk of infections.

Under what other circumstances would you consider breaking confidentiality?

- For notifiable diseases
- Where it is deemed to be in the public interest, e.g. threat of murder/terrorism
- Due to a court order
- Acting in the patient's best interests, e.g. if there are mental health issues or if the patient is in an unconscious state

What would you do if you subsequently find out that he has not informed DVLA?

If, despite attempts to persuade the patient to inform DVLA himself, this has not happened, then you would inform the patient (ideally in person and in writing) that you have a legal obligation to inform DVLA yourself.

What do you know about new agents used for the treatment of type II diabetes

See Station 2, p. 79.

Variations on the theme of fitness to drive

- Advising a newly diagnosed epileptic to stop driving

Tips

It is important to familiarize yourself with the DVLA guidelines for the common medical conditions e.g. epilepsy, diabetes, heart disease and dementia.

Case 7

Information for the candidate

You are the medical doctor. You are called by the ward nurse to speak to Miss Jones. She was admitted 48 hours ago with pyelonephritis and has improved with IV antibiotics. She is due for discharge on oral ciprofloxacin 500 mg b.d. However, during her admission, she was prescribed temazepam 10 mg o.n. by the on-call team since she complained she could not sleep. This was not included in her discharge medications. However, the ward nurse explains that Miss Jones is demanding to be discharged with a month's supply of temazepam 10 mg o.n. On review of the notes, Miss Jones is 39 years old, with no relevant past medical history. She is not on any regular medication.

Please speak to Miss Jones about prescribing her 1 month's supply of temazepam.

Brief for the actor

You are Daisy Jones, a 39-year-old lady who owns a café. For the past 8 weeks you have had trouble sleeping. This is becoming progressively worse and over the last 4 weeks you hardly slept, sleeping a maximum of 2–3 hours per night. When admitted to hospital recently for a kidney infection, the medical on-call prescribed you some sleeping tablets. You slept better. You have not used sleeping tablets in the past.

You own a café, and have been consumed by worry about the business. You have fallen into a lot of debt and worry the business could fold anytime soon. You are generally becoming more irritable. You live with your boyfriend. You lack interests. You are do not smoke or use recreational drugs. You drink 2–3 units of alcohol on special occasions. You may answer 'no' to any other questions posed about your psychological or physical wellbeing.

You have tried various simple measures to improve sleep such as leaving the room and reading. These have made little difference. The sleeping tablets in hospital were so useful that you want a supply for 1 month. You will become irritated with the doctor if asked other questions about work and personal circumstances.

If the doctor is sensitive and interested in your circumstances, you begin to open up and speak more freely about the situation. You will then recognize and accept that these factors are contributing to your sleep problems. However, you still want some sleeping tablets. If the doctor addresses your concerns about not sleeping and explains why he/she can only prescribe a short course of sleeping tablets, you find this acceptable. If the doctor does not address these issues, then you maintain your request for several weeks' supply.

Preparation

Make sure you appreciate the main points in the history:

- Establish the reason for requesting sleeping tablets

- Explore any measures she has taken to help her sleep
- Screen for anxiety and depression

Ethical and communication issues:

- Respect the patient's request even if you do not necessarily agree with it
- Be prepared to listen to the patient's reasons for requesting a month's supply of medication
- Ensure the patient is fully informed of the risks of taking long term courses of sleeping tablets
- Emphasize alternative courses of action in managing the sleep problem
- Be prepared to negotiate with the patient

Discussion with the patient

Introduction

- Introduce yourself
- Explain you were asked to speak to her by the ward nurse
- Clarify why Miss Jones wants sleeping tablets
- Exclude depression and suicidal risk

Provide an explanation

- Explain that you think the main factors affecting her sleep are related to the stressful situation surrounding her financial circumstances.

Discuss conservative measures

Sleep hygiene

- Go to bed and get up from bed at the same time each day
- Exercise regularly each day. Evidence suggests regular exercise improves restful sleep
- Get regular exposure to outdoor or bright lights, especially in the late afternoon
- The temperature in your bedroom should be comfortable
- Your bedroom should be dark enough to facilitate sleep
- Keep the bedroom as quiet as possible
- Use your bed only for sleep and sex
- Use relaxation exercises and breathing techniques prior to going to sleep
- Have a warm bath, massage or use balms to relax the muscles

Stress management

- Yoga
- Meditation
- Aromatherapy
- Exercise and hobbies

Offer support services

- Offer counselling CBT

- Suggest she seek help with her debts and finances, e.g. by speaking to her bank manager
- Inform her of support groups such as the Sleep Council and British Sleep Society

Consider medical treatments

- Explain that sleeping tablets are a short-term solution and do not address the root of the problem
- Highlight that if used long term could lead to dependence
- Discuss the side effects of sleeping tablets e.g. tiredness in the daytime and developing tolerance, Decline to offer a prescription or offer a short course for 3 days with follow up with her GP

Offer follow up

- Suggest she sees her GP to discuss her sleeping problems, further management and possible sick leave
- Provide her with information leaflets about insomnia

Discussion with the examiner

Potential areas of discussion include:

What do you know about insomnia?

- 1 in 5 people have some form of sleep disturbance.
- Females are affected > males and it is more common with age.
- Insomnia can be classified as primary or secondary.

Can you explain primary and secondary insomnia?

- Primary insomnia occurs when there are no associated underlying conditions.
- Secondary insomnia is associated with underlying conditions:
  - psychological illness e.g. bipolar disorder, depression and anxiety
  - physical illness e.g. sleep apnoea, asthma, hyperthyroidism, heart failure
  - drug use e.g. antidepressants, anti-epileptics, β-blockers, oral theophyllines and steroids

How do you manage patients with insomnia?

Short-term (<4 weeks) insomnia management

- Discuss sleep hygiene measures (also useful to discuss for long-term insomnia management)
- Consider a short course of sleeping tablets
  - advise the patient that sleeping tablets cannot be prescribed repeatedly
  - start at a low dose and warn about side effects
- If after 2 weeks the patient still has sleeping problems, consider cognitive–behavioural therapy (CBT).

Long-term (<4 weeks) insomnia management

Table 10 Management options in long-term insomnia

Relaxation therapies	Relaxation classes Audio material Meditation Breathing techniques
CBT	Re-train negative thoughts about falling asleep
Biofeedback	Trains the patient to control certain physiological processes e.g. heart rate, breathing rate and BP
Sleep restriction therapies	Patients are advised to restrict their sleeping hours so they eventually become tired again and establish new routines to fall asleep

- Avoid use of hypnotics for long-term insomnia except for acute relapses
- There is not enough evidence to support the use of antidepressants, antihistamines and barbiturates for insomnia. Antidepressants may be useful if there is underlying anxiety or depression.

When should a patient be referred to a sleep clinic?

- Consider referral to a sleep clinic in patients for:
  - primary insomnia
  - long-term insomnia not responding to treatment
  - patients where there is diagnostic uncertainty

Case 8

Information for the candidate

You are a medical doctor with the Dermatology team. You are reviewing Salima Shah, a 24-year-old Pakistani lady, who was referred to you by her GP with moles on her left thigh and right shoulder. She saw her GP because she was worried these could be cancerous and would like them removed. She has no family history of skin cancer, is on no regular medication and has no relevant past medical history. She seems quiet and when you offer to examine her she initially declines. However, you explain the necessity for the examination and she reluctantly accepts. Examination reveals two benign moles. However, you notice she has several bruises on her limbs, back and abdomen. You are worried she may be experiencing domestic violence. Please discuss this with the patient.

Brief for the actor

You are Salima Shah, a 24-year-old Pakistani lady. You noticed two moles on your left thigh and right shoulder. You saw your GP because you were worried these may be cancerous and want the moles removed. He referred you to the dermatology team to have them reviewed. You have come to the OPD alone because your husband, Khalid, was at work. He does not know you have attended today.

Two days ago Khalid became angry because you were on the telephone to your mother in Pakistan. He abused you because he did not want you to contact your family and calling Pakistan was too expensive. You tried to explain you called your mother because she had recently had hip surgery following a fall. He punched you on the arms several times, pushed you and then kicked you on your back and legs. He told you he would kill you if you 'misbehaved' again. You are terrified and unsure of what to do next, or who to speak to.

You lived in Pakistan and moved to the UK 6 months ago after having an arranged marriage. Khalid drinks heavily and when drunk he has forced you to have sex. You do not have children. Khalid refused to let you work. You have no friends in the UK. You are scared of leaving Khalid – you cannot support yourself financially and are concerned how your community will react if you did. You believe you will not be allowed to stay in the UK if you leave him, and will cause shame to your family if you return to Pakistan.

The violence occurs every few days. It happens at home. You have not spoken to anyone because you feel you are to blame. You are not suicidal but feel confused and scared. Khalid has never hit you with an object, or tried to strangle you. You have never called the police and are unaware of any services available to help you.

During the consultation, you appear timid. If the doctor asks you how the injury occurred, you say that you 'fell over'. If the doctor is caring and approaches the topic of domestic violence, you will open up slowly and explain how the injury really happened. You provide small amounts of information at first, but if the doctor shows empathy, you answer the questions with more detail. If the doctor communicates poorly, you stop talking or maintain the bruises occurred from falling over.

Preparation

Make sure you appreciate the main points

- Reassure the patient that the moles are benign and do not need to be removed
- Conduct a domestic violence risk assessment

Ethical and communication issues

- Use open body language and approach the situation in a gentle and non-threatening way
- Allow for silence, giving her time to speak
- Explore her fears about her marital situation
- Explore her cultural and religious beliefs about marriage
- Encourage her that she has options available
- Respect her autonomy on future action, and do not pressurize her into following a particular course of action

Discussion with the patient

Introduction

- Introduce yourself and explain you work for the dermatology team
- Reassure Salima that both moles are non-cancerous
- Explain the sinister features of moles e.g. bleeding, itching, growing in size and advise her to speak to her GP if these occur
- Sensitively discuss your suspicions of domestic violence as a cause of the bruises

Provide information

- Offer information sensitively, checking the patient's understanding as you go along
- Reassure her that confidentiality will be maintained
- Make it clear that the abuse is **not** her fault, and that 'violence in the home is illegal, just like violence on the street'
- Emphasize she is a victim of crime, has legal rights, and a right to safety
- Let her know she is not alone – 25% of women experience abuse
- Encourage her to see there is life after abuse – other women have created safer lives for themselves and so can she
- Discuss the physical and emotional consequences of chronic abuse
- Ask what **she** would like you to do, explaining agencies may be able to help where you cannot
- Provide written information about legal options and help offered by:
  - police domestic violence units
  - women's Aid National Helpline
  - local women's refuges and shelters
  - social service and local authority housing departments

*If children are involved, an urgent referral to the child protection team or social services is needed

Decide on a plan of action

- Respect her autonomy
- Explore the potential cultural reasons that prevent her from leaving her husband
- Discuss whether she wants to leave her partner, or stay with him
- If she wants to leave her partner, provide her with details on local services available, and offer help with contacting them
- If she chooses to return to her partner:
  - Give her the phone number of a local woman's refuge or the local Women's Aid
  - Advise her to keep some money and important financial and legal documents hidden in a safe place in case of an emergency
  - Advise her to avoid places such as the kitchen when the abuse starts, where there are potential weapons
  - Help her to plan an escape route in case of emergency
  - Educate her on calling 999 if needed. Advise her to tell a neighbour who can call 999 if they can hear the abuse

Follow-up

- Advise her to have follow up with her GP – offer to speak to her GP on her behalf and make an appointment for her

Discussion with the examiner

Potential areas of discussion include:

Tell me about domestic violence

- Domestic violence occurs in all parts of society, accounting for a quarter of all violent crime.
- Partner abuse is as common among same-sex couples as heterosexual couples.
- Particularly vulnerable groups are women with low socio-economic status or mental illness.
- Domestic violence is more likely to begin or escalate during pregnancy.
- If language is a barrier, remember always to use a professional interpreter, not a relative or friend.

How common is domestic violence?

- 2 women are killed every week by a current or former partner.
- 20% of women in England and Wales say they have been physically assaulted by their partner at some stage.
- 30% of domestic violence cases start during pregnancy.
- 52% of child protection cases involved domestic violence.
- 90% of domestic violence happens with the child or children in the same or next room.

*These are reported cases, therefore probably underestimate true figures

Can you give examples of domestic abuse?

- Physical abuse: shaking, smacking, punching, kicking, starving, tying up, stabbing, suffocation, throwing things, using objects as weapons and female genital mutilation.
- Sexual abuse: forced sex, forced prostitution, refusal to practise safe sex and sexual insults.
- Psychological abuse: intimidation, insulting, isolating the victim from friends and family, criticizing and treating the victim as an inferior.
- Financial abuse: not letting a woman work, undermining efforts to find work or study, refusing to give money, asking for an explanation of how every penny is spent and making her beg for money.
- Emotional abuse: swearing, undermining confidence, making racist remarks, making a woman feel unattractive, calling her stupid or useless and eroding her independence.

What are the effects of domestic abuse?

Table 11 The physical and psychological effects of domestic violence

Physical effects	Psychological effects
Death	Suicide
Bruising	Self-harming behaviour
Tiredness	Fear
Poor nutrition	Guilt
Broken bones	Depression
Chronic pain	Post-traumatic stress disorder
Miscarriage	Increased misuse of drugs and alcohol
Maternal death	Loss of self-confidence
Premature birth	Loss of hope
Babies with low birth weight or stillborn	Low self-worth
General poor health	Panic or anxiety
Burns or stab wounds	Eating disorders

What service can you signpost this patient too?

- Free phone 24-hour National Domestic Violence Helpline (0808 2000 247).
- This runs in partnership with women's aid and refuge.
- Provides information, emotional and practical support to women.
- Calls are taken in confidence.
- Also consider referral to refuge and outreach services.

Case 9

Information for the candidate

You are the junior doctor in the general medical outpatient clinic. Mrs Angi O'Gram is a 64-year old lady who is attending a follow up appointment. Your consultant saw her 2 weeks ago and confirmed she has multiple myeloma. At the time she was extremely distraught, so management options were only briefly discussed. Your consultant decided to allow her some time to come to terms with the diagnosis and to come back 2 weeks later to explore management options. In that time an MDT meeting has been held which concluded that the best treatment would be chemotherapy and steroids and that this should be implemented as soon as possible. She is here to see you to discuss management options.

Brief for the actor

You are Angi O'Gram, a 64-year old lady. Two weeks ago you were diagnosed with a type of cancer called multiple myeloma. This came as a shock to you and you were too upset to discuss management options. The consultant mentioned it is likely that you will require steroids and chemotherapy. Today you feel calmer. You have spent a lot of time discussing further management with your family. You have also spent a lot of time reading about chemotherapy on the internet. You were scared to learn that chemotherapy can make your hair fall out and cause infections. You are also very worried about the prospects of taking steroids as you have also read up in their side effects, particularly of weight gain and high BP. In your research you have also read a lot about homeopathy and have spoken to a friend who says it cured them of cancer (you do not know which type). You feel that this would provide hope of a cure and avoid the side effects of western treatments. Your main agenda going to this consultation is that you want a referral to see a homeopathic specialist because you believe this will provide you with the best hope of a cure. You spoke to your GP who refused to refer you, but you read on the internet that The Royal London Hospital for integrated medicine accepts referrals directly from the NHS hospital consultants. If the doctor is sympathetic and explains the benefits of chemotherapy and steroids well, as well addressing concerns about side effects then you may be persuaded to approach their suggestions.

Preparation

Make sure you appreciate the main points

- Without the right treatment myeloma has a poor prognosis
- The patient favours an alternative therapy that is unlikely to provide a cure for myeloma
- Respect the patient's views about conventional therapies and be prepared to discuss the benefits and risks of chemotherapy and steroids

Ethical and communication issues

- Approach the case with sensitivity and compassion
- Be prepared to listen to the patient's views about alternative treatments and the research she has carried out
- Ensure the patient is provided with informed consent about the pros and cons of proposed treatments

Discussion with the patient

Introduction

- Introduce yourself

Check the patient's understanding of myeloma and her proposed option

- Explore her understanding of this condition and of homeopathy
- Emphasize the serious nature of this condition, explaining that without treatment myeloma has a poorer prognosis with a substantially reduced life expectancy

Discussion of management options

- Highlight that myeloma may be incurable, but that current treatments are available to control the disease, maximize quality of life and prolong survival

- Explain that using chemotherapy and steroids significantly improves her chances of survival
- Explain that there is no evidence to suggest homeopathy alone is a curative treatment for myeloma or improves survival
- Emphasize that time is a limiting factor – the longer the cancer is left untreated, the more likely she is to have an adverse outcome
- Supportive measures include:
  - blood transfusion for anaemia
  - antibiotics for bacterial infection
  - radiotherapy to treat localized painful lesions
- Explain the role of the multidisciplinary team in supporting her, including the GP, palliative care nurses and oncologists

Address the patient's concerns about chemotherapy and steroids

- Discuss the common side effects of chemotherapy and steroid treatment, particularly addressing the ones that concern her most:

Alopecia

- Inform her many people go on to wear wigs, hats and scarves
- Explain this is a temporary effect and hair will grow back a few months after stopping treatment

Other

- Discuss the side effects of steroids, informing her that complications such as hypertension and type 2 diabetes are less common with short-term steroid treatment which is what she would require
- Reassure her that her BP and blood sugar will be monitored to manage these complications if they develop
- Explain that side effects such as nausea and vomiting can be well controlled with medication

Agree an action plan before the consultation ends

- The ideal outcome would be to try and persuade the patient to agree to your suggested treatment
- This might mean agreeing to a homeopathy referral alongside conventional treatment as a compromise
- Arrange referral to a haematologist/oncologist and organize follow-up

Discussion with the examiner

Potential areas of discussion include:

Tell me about homeopathy

- Homeopathy works on the theory 'like cures like'. The homeopathic substance is highly diluted.
- The more diluted the substance, the greater its potency. Many of the substances come from plants.

- Homeopathy's main practical use is for self-limiting conditions e.g. hay fever, influenza and vertigo.
- There is no evidence to suggest that homeopathy can cure cancer.
- It should not be used to treat harmful diseases where there is not enough evidence to support its benefits.

What are the homeopathic centres in the UK?

- The Royal London Hopsital for Integrated Medicine
- Glasgow Homeopathic Hospital
- Bristol Homeopathic Hospital
- Liverpool Medical Homeopathy Service

What is myeloma?

- This is a malignancy of plasma cells within the bone marrow.
- It results in a clonal expansion of plasma cells which produce a monoclonal paraprotein, mostly IgG.
- There is often excretion of light chains within the urine, so called Bence–Jones proteins.

Who does this usually affect?

- The most likely affected groups are:
  - patients >60 years of age
  - males
  - black Africans

What are the main features of myeloma?

- Bone marrow destruction, leading to anaemia, neutropenia, thrombocytopenia and paraproteinaemia
- Renal failure
- Hypercalcaemia
- Bone destruction

How would you diagnose myeloma?

The diagnosis can be made with two out the three of the following:

- Paraproteinaemia or Bence–Jones protein
- Lytic bone lesions on X-ray
- Raised plasma cell levels within the bone marrow

Briefly outline the mainstay of treatment in myeloma

- Treat complications, for example anaemia, recurrent infections and bone pain.
- Specific treatments:
  - these remain palliative
  - chemotherapy and steroids remain the main treatment. Examples of chemotherapeutic agents include melphalan, vincristine and thalidomide
  - combination of chemotherapy and autologous stem cell transplant can also be used

What do you know about the prognosis of myeloma?

- The international prognostic index helps assess this. It is based on the serum albumin and β_2 microglobulin:

Stage	β_2 microglobulin	Serum albumin	Median survival (months)
1	< 3.5 mg/L	≥ 35 g/L	62 months
2	Not stage 1 or 3	Not stage 1 or 3	44 months
3	≥ 5.5 mg/L	–	29 months

- Overall prognosis, with access to medical care, is a 5-year median survival (occasionally up to 10 years).

1

STATION 5 INTEGRATED CLINICAL ASSESSMENT

Case 1

Information for the candidate

Your role: you are one of the medical doctors on a ward round.
Patient details: Mrs Sarah Green, aged 35 years.
This lady was admitted with pyelonephritis and is ready for discharge today. She mentions to you that over the past 6 months she has experienced episodes of blurry vision in her right eye.
Your task: to address the patient's problems and any questions or concerns raised.

Information for the patient

You are: Mrs Green, aged 35 years.
Your problem: over the past 6 months you have experienced episodes of blurry vision in the right eye.
You have been in hospital with a kidney infection for 3 days; this has now settled with IV antibiotics and you now feel back to normal. The medical doctor is about to review you on the ward round, hopefully to send you home.

Up until now, you believed that the blurred vision would go away and therefore did not approach any doctors. If asked, the episodes have increased in frequency. They now occur every couple of days and last for up to 30 minutes. The symptoms are beginning to frustrate you, particularly because they can come on at any time, e.g. at work when you are on the computer or in a meeting.

If asked, you have not experienced any pain, loss of sensation, weakness, limb paralysis, headaches, or loss of consciousness.

Apart from this latest kidney infection, you are otherwise fit and well. Your only treatment is the oral contraceptive pill. You work as a secretary in the city. You are married with no children. You smoke five cigarettes a day. If asked, there are no significant illnesses running in the family. You have two brothers and one sister, all fit and well. Both your parents are alive and well.
You should ask: what the doctor thinks is wrong. You are worried about going blind and wonder if that is a possibility. You are wondering what needs to be done to look into and treat this.

Clinical consultation

In the 8 minutes with the patient, the candidate would be expected to:

- Take a detailed history of the visual disturbances – this should include asking how long Mrs Green sits staring at the computer screen and whether she has had an eye check for refractive problems
- Demonstrate that you are thinking of the key differentials (listed below)
- Enquire about medical history, drug history and occupational history, particularly any chemical exposures e.g. lead
- Examine the eyes, including fundoscopy
- Explain the need for carrying out blood tests, checking intraocular pressures and urgent referral to an ophthalmologist

Discussion with the examiner

In the 2 minutes for discussion, the candidate might be asked:

What are the potential causes of blurred vision?

Ocular

- Trauma
- Cataract
- Lens refraction problems
- Glaucoma
- Uveitis
- Optic neuritis. e.g. MS
- Retinal detachment
- Diabetic retinopathy
- Central retinal vein occlusion
- Central retinal artery occlusion
- Macular degeneration

Other

- Migraine
- Temporal arteritis
- Space-occupying lesion
- Vascular event – TIA, CVA, bleed

You will be guided by what is found on examination. In this particular case we are focusing on optic atrophy as the cause of the patient's loss of vision. However be aware that the exam may focus on one of the other potential causes above.

Describe any abnormal clinical findings

On examination of the fundi, there are pale and well-defined optic discs. There is also a relative afferent pupillary defect (RAPD), whereby the pupil reacts to light consensually but not directly. I would like to check this patient's vision, which may show a central scotoma.

The patient has optic atrophy (Figure 4). My main differential in this case would be optic neuritis. I would also like to perform a full neurological examination to determine if this patient has multiple sclerosis.

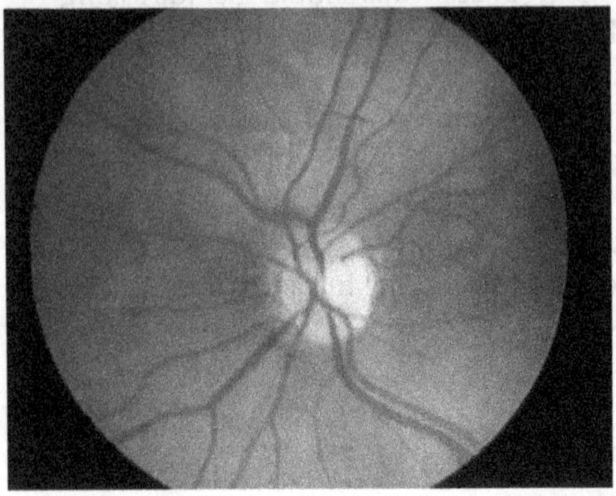

Figure 4 Optic atrophy. Reproduced with permission of Omar Malik.

What is the difference between optic neuritis and optic atrophy?

- Optic neuritis occurs when the optic nerve is inflamed and the disc is swollen. The disc may look normal or swollen.
- Optic atrophy can occur as a late sign when the demyelination has occurred and the disc shrunk back.
- The most common cause for optic neuritis is multiple sclerosis.
- Optic neuritis may present with visual symptoms, pain and disturbance in colour vision (which the patient might not have realized until asked or tested).

What are the features of optic nerve damage?

- RAPD
- Optic atrophy
- Central scotoma
- Decreased visual acuity
- Reduced colour vision

What are the common causes of optic atrophy?

Systemic causes

- Multiple sclerosis – commonest cause
- Friedreich's ataxia
- Paget's disease
- Vitamin B_{12} deficiency
- Toxins such as alcohol, lead, tobacco and cyanide
- Infections such as syphilis, toxoplasmosis and CMV
- Frontal brain tumour
    - known as Foster–Kennedy syndrome
    - papilloedema found in one eye due to raised intracranial pressure
    - optic atrophy in the other eye due to direct compression by the tumour

Ocular causes

- Glaucoma
- Leber's optic atrophy
- Retinitis pigmentosa
- Central retinal artery occlusion

How would you manage this case?

- Arrange blood tests – vitamin B_{12}, iron studies, glucose
- MRI of brain
- Arrange urgent ophthalmology referral
- The patient can go home in the meantime

Case 2

Information for the candidate

Your role: you are the medical doctor in outpatients.
Patient details: Mr Smith, aged 55 years.
This gentleman was referred by his GP with a rash on the shins for 4 weeks. The referral letter also mentions the presence of a lesion on the nose, which has been present for 3 months.
Your task: review the patient and address any questions or concerns that may arise.

Information for the patient

You are: Mr Smith, aged 55 years
Your problem: painful rash on the shins for 1 month and unsightly rash on the nose for 3 months.
The rash on the shins came on gradually. Initially you went to the GP who prescribed ibuprofen. This helped the pain but the rash has spread on the shins and does not seem to be settling. The rash on the nose is not painful and not itchy. There are no obvious underlying triggers for these problems. You have no other significant medical history other than mild asthma. You occasionally use a ventolin inhaler for mild breathlessness upon exercise but you have no cough and no wheeze. You are on no other prescribed medications except for ibuprofen.

If asked, you have no bowel symptoms, no weight loss, and no eye symptoms. You can answer 'no' to any other symptoms you are asked about. You have had no recent travel abroad.

You are married with two children who are both at university. You work as an accountant. You are a lifelong non-smoker and drink 10 units of alcohol per week.
You should ask: why you have the skin rash on the shins and nose. You would also like to know what needs to be done to treat it.

Clinical consultation

In the 8 minutes with the patient, the candidate would be expected to:

- Obtain a detailed history
- Rule out potential causes for erythema nodosum (see causes listed below)

- Examine the shins and nose
- Explain to the patient findings of erythema nodosum and lupus pernio
- Share your working diagnosis with the patient as well as the need to perform blood tests and a CXR

Discussion with the examiner

In the 2 minutes for discussion, the candidate might be asked:

Explain your examination findings

The lesions on the shins are raised, nodular, erythematous and tender (they can sometimes also present on the forearms). This is consistent with erythema nodosum (Figure 5).

On the nose, there are reddish-purple plaques. I would also like to check for these on the hands, feet and ears. This patient has lupus pernio.

These findings are consistent with a diagnosis of sarcoidosis. I would like to examine the eyes for signs of uveitis and the chest for signs of respiratory sarcoid.

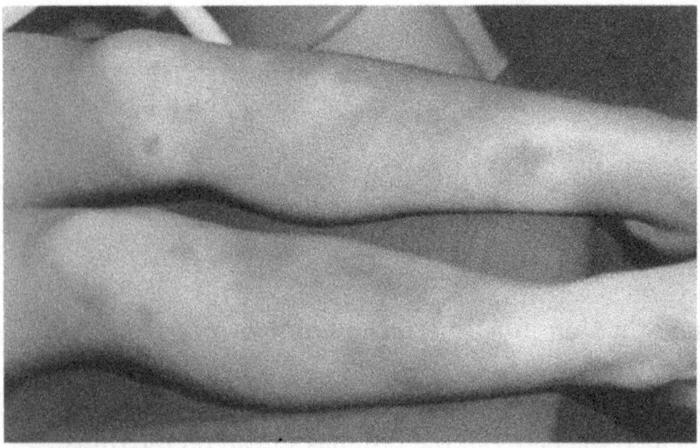

Figure 5 Erythema nodosum. Reproduced with permission of Aruna Dias from *Get Through MRCP Part 2: 350 Best of Fives*. London: RSM Press.

Why do you think this patient has sarcoidosis?

He has a combination of erythema nodosum and lupus pernio.

What are the possible causes of erythema nodosum?

- Infections – streptococcal, TB
- Sarcoidosis
- Drugs – oral contraceptive, sulfonamides, penicillin, salicylates
- Pregnancy
- Inflammatory bowel disease
- Rheumatic fever
- Neoplastic disease, e.g. lymphoma
- Other infections – syphilis, leprosy, toxoplasmosis, *Yersinia* spp., fungal infections (e.g. tinea)

How would you manage erythema nodosum?

Supportive

- Bed rest
- Local treatment (compresses)

Medical

- NSAIDs – often settles with these alone
- Steroid therapy (infrequently used)
- Treat underlying cause

What are the clinical features of erythema nodosum?

- Fever
- Malaise
- Arthralgia
- The lesions usually disappear within 6 weeks

What might lupus pernio be confused with?

- Rhinophyma
- SLE
- Rosacea

What treatment is used for lupus pernio?

- Topical or intralesional steroids
- Oral steroids or immunosuppressive therapy if the patient has systemic sarcoid

What are the skin manifestations of sarcoidosis?

- Erythema nodosum
- Papules
- Plaques
- Subcutaneous nodules
- Keloid scars
- Lupus pernio

Discuss the investigations you wish to perform in this patient and any further management

- Blood tests:
  - FBC
  - ESR/CRP
  - calcium levels
  - ASO titres
  - serum ACE
  - syphilis serology
- Throat swab
- CXR – for hilar lymphadenopathy

- Consider dermatology input for skin biopsy of the nose to confirm non-caseating granulomas
- Arrange follow-up and referral to respiratory physician

Case 3

Information for the candidate

Your role: you are the medical doctor on call.
Patient details: Mr A Jones, aged 50 years.
This gentleman has presented to the casualty department complaining of double vision.
Your task: assess the patient's problems and answer any questions he has.

Information for the patient

You are: Mr A Jones, aged 50 years.
Your problem: For the past 2 weeks you have experienced worsening episodes of double vision (which you think are coming from the left eye).
There are no obvious triggers for this. There is no pain. You have also noticed that it is harder to open the left eye.

Your only medical history is well-controlled hypertension which was diagnosed 5 years ago. Your last BP check a month ago (at the GP) showed that it was under control. You currently take Ramipril 5 mg o.d. You are on no other medications and have no other significant medical history. If asked, your father also suffered from hypertension and died of a heart attack, aged 70. He was diagnosed with type II diabetes in his sixties. There is no other significant family history.

You work as a car salesperson. You are married with two children. You are a former smoker of 10 cigarettes a day and gave up 10 years ago.
You should ask: what is wrong, why you have double vision and check if everything will be okay.

Clinical consultation

In the 8 minutes with the patient, the candidate will be expected to:

- Obtain a detailed history
- Appreciate that a neurosurgical cause needs to be ruled out
- Appreciate that the history of hypertension could be clinically relevant and make a focused enquiry about this and cardiac risk factors
- Perform a targeted eye examination demonstrating the key abnormalities
- Explain the need for an urgent MRI scan to rule out surgical causes.

Discussion with the examiner

In the 2 minutes for discussion, the candidate could be asked:

Describe your clinical findings

On examination there is ptosis of the left eye (due to the paralysis of levator palpebrae superioris). There is a divergent strabismus. The pupil is fixed in a down and out position (due to the unopposed action of lateral rectus and superior oblique). It is dilated and reacts slowly to light. The patient has diplopia which is worse when looking to the left side. The outer image disappears when the left eye is covered.

This patient has a CN III palsy affecting the left eye.

Broadly outline the main causes for double vision

Binocular double vision

- Brain tumour
- Multiple sclerosis
- Myasthenia gravis
- Thyroid eye disease
- Vascular disease/CVA
- Aneurysm
- Head injury

Monocular double vision

- Astigmatism
- Cataract (rare)
- Eye lens dislocation
- Dry eyes
- Eyelid pathology, e.g. swelling

What are the causes of a CN III palsy?

- A CN III palsy can result from intrinsic (medical) causes due to microvascular damage, or extrinsic (surgical) compression by aneurysm or tumour.
- In medical lesions, ophthalmoplegia is the predominant clinical sign. The ptosis or pupil dilation signs are mild.
- In surgical lesions the ptosis and pupil dilation are the predominant signs. The ophthalmoplegia is minimal. This is because the parasympathetic nerves, which are responsible for pupil constriction, run on the outside of CN III. These are affected by external compression, leading to an inability to constrict the pupil, which is thus dilated.

Medical causes

- Hypertension
- Mononeuritis multiplex
- Midbrain demyelination
- Myasthenia gravis
- Weber's syndrome: CN III palsy with contralateral hemiplegia

Surgical causes

- Aneurysm of the posterior communicating artery
- Cavernous sinus thrombosis, fistula or tumour
- Cerebral uncus herniation

- NB: Raised intracranial pressure can present as a CN III palsy. This would be a false localizing sign.

What are the causes of a mononeuritis multiplex?

- Diabetes
- Carcinoma
- Amyloidosis
- Sarcoidosis
- Lyme disease
- Leprosy
- HIV
- PAN
- Rheumatoid arthritis
- SLE
- Churg–Strauss syndrome
- Sjögren's syndrome
- Wegener's granulomatosis

What cranial nerves innervate the eye muscles?

- Oculomotor (CN III): superior, inferior and medial rectus muscles
- Inferior oblique
- Trochlear (CN IV): superior oblique
- Abducens (CN VI): lateral rectus

How would you manage this patient?

- Investigation of medical causes
- MRI of brain
- Neurosurgical referral if aneurysm or cerebral mass identified

Describe what you might see on examination in a patient with a CN VI palsy

On examination, the head is turned laterally towards the left side (same side as the paralysed muscle) in order to neutralize diplopia. The left eye is deviated medially and there is impairment of lateral movement. Diplopia is worse on looking to the left. The outer image disappears when the left eye is covered.

This patient has a CN VI palsy.

What are the causes of a CN VI palsy?

- Hypertension
- Multiple sclerosis
- Diabetes
- Mononeuritis multiplex
- Myasthenia gravis
- Cerebrovascular accidents
- Trauma such as fractured base of skull
- Raised intracranial pressure (false localizing sign) due to space-occupying lesion

Case 4

Information for the candidate

Your role: you are the medical doctor on call.
Patient details: Mr Michael Miller, aged 38 years.

He was admitted to the ENT ward for an elective removal of nasal polyps for recurrent nosebleeds. The ENT doctors discovered that he had some red macules on the lips and they have now asked for a medical opinion. Your consultant asks you to review this patient.
Your task: assess the patient's problem and address any questions and concerns he has.

Information for the patient

You are: Mr Michael Miller, aged 38 years.
Your problem: you have been admitted to an ENT ward for a routine operation to have some nasal polyps removed. One of the junior doctors on the ward noted that you had small spots on the lips and said they might be part of an underlying condition, which could explain the nosebleeds.

You have in the past had several attendances to casualty for nosebleeds and required nasal packing to terminate these bleeds. The history of nosebleeds dates back to childhood. They have recently become more frequent. The ENT specialists identified several nasal polyps which they think are probably the cause. You have now been admitted to have these removed.

If asked about the spots on your lips, you have had these spots ever since you can remember and did not think they were anything worrying. Your partner commented that they seem to be more pronounced recently. You also noticed some rashes on the face.

If asked, your only medical history is a chest infection you had 5 years ago which required two courses of antibiotics by your GP. You did experience blood in the sputum at that time but this settled within a week. You were found to be mildly anaemic following some of the nosebleeds in the past but your doctor told you this had now settled. You are on no prescribed medication.

Your father passed away previously following a large gastrointestinal bleed. Your sister also suffers from nosebleeds but these have been relatively minor, not requiring surgery.
You should ask: the reason for the nosebleeds and an explanation for the spots on your lips.

Clinical consultation

In the 8 minutes with the patient, the candidate should:

- Obtain a detailed history – including the nosebleeds and enquiry about the skin lesions on the lips (particularly worth examining while taking the history)
- Enquire about a history of any other bleeds – including gastrointestinal/pulmonary; ask about iron deficiency anaemia
- Ask about family history, appreciating that this condition might follow an autosomal dominant pattern of inheritance
- Examine the nose, lips, face and palate for further lesions
- Explain the possible link between the skin lesions and nosebleeds and the need to investigate for this. Also, make a brief mention about genetic screening.

Discussion with the examiner

In the 2 minutes for discussion, the candidate might be asked:

Explain your examination findings

There are red macules on the lips and papules on the face that blanch on pressure. I would also like to examine the tongue, palate and fingers as well as to look for signs of anaemia.

These skin lesions are telangiectasia.

If you pick up signs of anaemia, which condition do you think this patient has?

Hereditary haemorrhagic telangiectasia

Is this an inherited condition?

Yes, it is autosomal dominant

What are the complications of this condition?

- Gastrointestinal bleeds causing iron deficiency anaemia (due to telangiectasia in the gastrointestinal tract)
- Epistaxis
- Haemoptysis
- Arteriovenous malformations: pulmonary, cerebral, hepatic

How would you manage a patient with this condition?

- Treat complications discussed above
- Patients often require iron replacement therapy due to chronic blood loss
- Genetic counselling

Case 5

Information for the candidate

Your role: you are the medical doctor in the rheumatology clinic.
Patient details: Mrs T Maitland, aged 35 years.
Your next patient has been referred in by the GP with a recent onset of back pain. Of note she has a long-standing history of psoriasis, which is being managed by the dermatology team.
Your task: assess the patient's problems and address any questions and concerns she may have.

Information for the patient

You are: Mrs T Maitland, aged 35 years.
Your problem: back pain.
You have had low back pain which has been worsening over the past 6 months. The pain tends to improve slightly with movement and get worse when sitting in one position. Recently you have been waking frequently at night with the pain and experiencing morning stiffness. Your GP prescribed you ibuprofen which helped initially but now has minimal effect. The pain is now present all the time.

You work as a manager for a local supermarket and the pain is beginning to interfere with your work. You usually play squash but this is no longer possible.

You have suffered from psoriasis for 5 years. This occurs in patches on the elbows, and shins. You are currently using topical treatments but in the past have received a course of PUVA therapy. You are currently under the management of the dermatologists and last saw them 2 months ago. The condition is currently stable. You may answer 'no' to any other clinical questions asked.

You should ask: what might be wrong with your back and what needs to be done.

Clinical consultation

In the 8 minutes with the patient, the candidate should cover the following:

- Detailed history about the problem – enquire about red flags, e.g. bladder/bowel symptoms, weight loss
- Appreciate the difference between mechanical and inflammatory back pain
- Enquire about the psoriasis – including treatments received (topical, UV therapy, disease-modifying agents), specialist involvement, how it affects her life and social history
- Examine the skin and back – offer to perform a neurological examination of the lower limbs
- Explain the need for blood tests, radiographs and possibly MRI scanning.

Discussion with the examiner

In the 2 minutes to discuss the case, the candidate might be asked:

Describe your examination findings

The patient has well-defined salmon pink plaques on her right shin. There are also plaques located on the extensor surfaces of the elbow. The nails and scalp are unremarkable. I would ideally like to check the entire body for other signs of psoriasis. The patient has psoriasis.

Upon examination of the back, there is a mild kyphosis but no other obvious deformity of the spine. There is limited flexion of the back to 60 degrees. Upon palpation there is tenderness in the sacroiliac region.

Taken together, these findings suggest this patient has a sacroileitis in the presence of psoriasis. I would also like to examine the lower limbs and to check for sacral anaesthesia and reduced anal sphincter tone.

What do you know about psoriatic arthropathy?

- Psoriatic arthritis belongs to a group of conditions that cause inflammation of the ligaments, tissues and synovium (spondyloarthropathies).
- It is a seronegative (RF negative) disease.
- It is an HLA-associated autoimmune disease. Patients often have HLA-B27.
- Males and females are equally affected
- It usually occurs in the fourth and fifth decades of life.
- Skin and joint disease can appear together or separately.

- Approximately 10% of patients with skin disease develop joint disease.
- Patients with psoriatic arthritis can develop inflammation of tendons, cartilage, eyes, lung lining and, rarely, the aorta.

What are the patterns of joint disease in psoriasis?

- **Asymmetrical oligo- or monoarthopathy:** affects up to five joints on different sides of the body such as one knee and a few finger joints
- **Symmetrical polyarthritis:** clinically indistinguishable from rheumatoid arthritis
- **Distal joint involvement:** affecting distal interphalangeal joints (IPJs) of fingers or toes
- **Arthritis mutilans:** severe arthritis of the distal IPJs leads to telescoping of the phalanges causing 'opera glass' deformities
- **Spondylitic pattern ± sacroileitis:** similar to ankylosing spondylitis but the vertebrae are usually affected asymmetrically

How would you investigate the patient in this case?

Bloods
- ESR and CRP may be elevated
- RF and ANA are negative
- HLA-B27 positive

Radiography
- Mild bony erosion at edge of cartilage
- Asymmetrical erosive changes in small joints of hands and feet
- Erosion of distal tuft of distal phalanx
- Classic pencil in cup appearance of distal IPJs in the presence of arthritis mutilans

MRI scan
- To rule out structural deformity or space-occupying lesion

What treatment options are available for patients with psoriatic arthropathy?

General
- Education
- Physiotherapy

Medical treatment
- NSAIDs for pain relief and treatment of swelling
- Intra-articular steroid injections for joint flare-ups
- Immunosuppressant drugs such as methotrexate, azathioprine, hydroxyurea, sulfasalazine, gold, penicillamine and ciclosporin can be used
- Etanercept and infliximab are useful to treat patients in whom DMARDs have failed

Surgical treatment
- For deformed joints to improve function

What are the various types of psoriasis?

- Plaque psoriasis – commonest type, as in this patient
- Guttate psoriasis – small spots over the body (Figure 6)
- Pustular psoriasis – pustules
- Flexural psoriasis
- Nail psoriasis
- Joint psoriasis (psoriatic arthropathy)

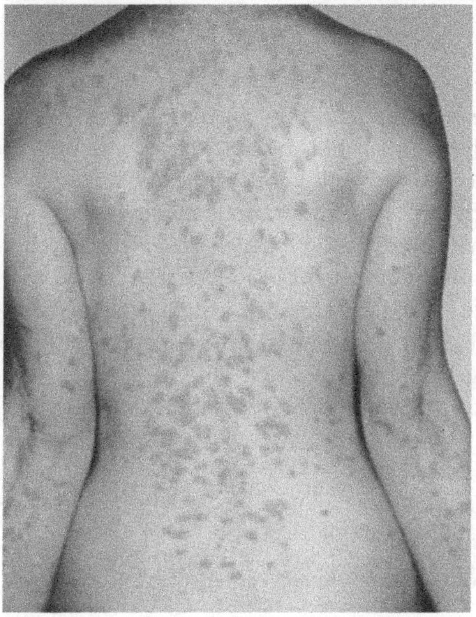

Figure 6 Guttate psoriasis. Reproduced with permission of Aruna Dias from *Get Through MRCP Part 2: 350 Best of Fives*. London: RSM Press.

What are the treatment options for psoriasis?

Supportive
- Education
- Psychological support

Topical
- Vitamin D_3 analogues
- Coal tar
- Dithranol
- Salicylic acid

Systemic
- Narrow band UVB/PUVA
- Immunosuppressive drugs, e.g. methotrexate, azathioprine, ciclosporin
- Hydroxyurea
- Biological agents

Case 6

Information for the candidate

Your role: you are the medical doctor in the general medical clinic.
Patient details: Mr John Benjamin, aged 42 years.
This gentleman presents to the clinic because the GP is concerned that he may have neurofibromatosis.
Your task: assess the patient's problems and address any concerns or questions he has.

Information for the patient

You are: Mr John Benjamin, aged 42 years.
Your problem: you have noted an increase in lumps in the skin and nodules. These have been present from your early teen years but you note that they have worsened over the past few years. If asked, you have also noticed freckles under the armpits. You have had several lipomas removed from various sites over the years. You have been told by your GP that your BP is on the high side. He has been keeping an eye on it over the past few months but you have not yet been started on any treatment for it. You were adopted and do not know your family history. At school you were a slow learner and did not do well at exams. You work at a petrol station and are married with two young children.
You should ask: why the GP has referred you and if there is something seriously wrong.

Clinical consultation

In the 8 minutes with the patient, the candidate should:

- Take a focused history, enquiring about the key features of neurofibromatosis in a systematic manner
- Appreciate that this condition is inherited by taking a family history
- Examine the patient – in the short space of time the key features to examine would mainly be those that you might find on inspection. Emphasize the importance of the skin lesions e.g. café-au-lait patches and neurofibromas
- Explain in simple terms what neurofibromatosis is, the tests required to confirm it and raise the issue of genetic counselling

Discussion with the examiner

In the 2 minutes to discuss the case, the candidate might be asked:

What is your diagnosis and why?

Neurofibromatosis, as evidenced by multiple neurofibromas and café-au-lait spots (more than five lesions is significant), as well as axillary freckling. I would like to examine the patient further to elicit any further manifestations of the disease (listed below).

Describe all the features you might find on inspection and palpation of a patient with this condition

- Neurofibromata and nodules felt along peripheral nerves
- Multiple lipomas

- Cutaneous fibromata
- Kyphoscoliosis
- Muscle wasting

What are the complications of this condition not already mentioned?

Central nervous system
- Cord compression
- Acoustic neuroma
- Meningioma
- Medulloblastomas
- Epilepsy

Peripheral nervous system – pressure effects of neurofibroma on peripheral nerves causing:
- Motor or sensory neuropathy
- Plexiform neuroma

Eyes
- Lisch nodules
- Optic glioma
- Retinal harmatomas

Musculoskeletal effects
- Dysplasias of bone (e.g. bowing of legs)
- Rib notching

Other
- Sarcomas
- Leukaemia (especially in children)
- Lung fibrosis
- Hypertension
- Learning disability (common problem)

Note: Lisch nodules are yellow–brown nodular lesions present on the iris, usually detected on slit lamp examination. Presence of café-au-lait patches, neurofibromas and Lisch nodules is highly suggestive of neurofibromatosis.

Discuss the various types of this condition

Table 12 Neurofibromatosis

	Type I	Type II
Inheritance	Autosomal dominant	Autosomal dominant
Affected chromosome	17	22
Signs	Café-au-lait spots Neurofibromas (mainly plexiform type) Axillary freckling Lisch nodules	Bilateral CN VIII neuromas More commonly central tumours
Other		Hearing tests for family members

How would you manage this condition?

- Management for both conditions is to treat complications as they occur
- Most patients are asymptomatic and require no treatment
- Genetic counselling for patients and family members

Case 7

Information for the candidate

Your role: you are the medical doctor in outpatients.
Patient details: Mrs Tracy Fellows, aged 28 years.
This lady was admitted to the gynaecology ward for an elective hysteroscopy for heavy periods. The procedure was uneventful and a small polyp was found. She also has epilepsy and the gynaecology team have asked for a medical opinion because she mentioned she has been having more fits lately.

Your consultant has asked you to review the patient.

Information for the patient

You are: Mrs Tracy Fellows, aged 28 years.
Your problem: increased seizures.
You are on the gynaecology ward having just had a hysteroscopic examination. You have epilepsy and you told one of the junior staff on the ward that you have experienced increased fits recently. These tend to involve jerking movements of the legs and arms and last for between 3 and 5 minutes. For the last 3 months, your fit frequency has been 2–3 per week, having previously been 1–2 per month. The episodes are sometimes associated with tongue biting but only occasionally have you had leaking of faeces or urine.

You have a known history of epilepsy and an inherited condition called tuberous sclerosis. You are currently taking sodium valproate. You have some associated skin conditions which include a rash on the face. If asked, your mother and brother both have the same medical conditions. As far as you are aware you have no other complications. You work in a library. You were always behind at school and did not complete your GCSE exams.
You should ask: if the fits are related to your condition and what needs to be done.

Clinical consultation

In the 8 minutes with the patient, the candidate should:

- Take a history of the fits – including details of the kinds of seizures, complications, fit frequency, treatments
- Elicit the past history of tuberous sclerosis and its previous history
- Enquire about social history, concerns and how her condition affects her
- Acknowledge the complications of tuberous sclerosis
- Examine the skin and nails to demonstrate the key skin features of tuberous sclerosis as well as offering to perform a full neurological examination
- Explain to the patient that epilepsy is a feature of tuberous sclerosis, the fits ought to be investigated with blood tests and possibly a CT/MRI scan, and that you will ask for an opinion from her specialist.

Discussion with the examiner

In the 2 minutes to discuss the case, the candidate might be asked:

Describe the lesions on this patient's face

There is a red, nodular eruption on the face, particularly in the butterfly distribution and in nasolabial folds. This is known as adenoma sebaceum. I would like to check for subungal fibroma, shagreen patches (leathery lesions on the low back) and ash-leaf patches (hypopigmented patches).

What do you think is the reason for the patient's seizures?

Tuberous sclerosis. The likelihood of this is increased by confirming the combination of adenoma sebaceum, low IQ and epilepsy.

What are the main features in the history that support this?

- History of epilepsy
- Family history of the same condition
- Learning difficulty in childhood

What investigations would you carry out?

- Bloods:
    - U&Es
    - glucose
    - calcium
    - FBC
    - LFTs
- Consider imaging (liaise with neurology)

How would you treat a patient with tuberous sclerosis?

- Offer genetic counselling
- Treat complications – for example, epilepsy (as in this case)

Describe other features of this condition

- Autosomal dominant (80%) or due to mutational changes (20%)
- Angiofibroma (adenoma sebaceum)
- Harmartomas in the CNS, kidney, retina, heart (rhabdomyomata)
- Cystic lesions (due to harmartomas) in lung, pancreas, kidney

What are the phakomatosis disorders and state some examples

- These are a group of over 20 neurocutanous syndromes. These conditions lead to phakomas (hamartomas) which exert pressure effects in various organs, mainly CNS, spinal cord and lung. They also predispose to malignancy. Examples include:
    - Tuberous sclerosis
    - Neurofibromatosis types I and II
    - Sturge–Weber syndrome

- Von Hippel–Lindau disease
- Ataxic telangiectasia

Sturge–Weber syndrome

- Sturge–Weber syndrome (encephalotrigeminal angiomatosis) is another phakoma that might present in the PACES exam. Questions that might be asked are outlined below.

How might a patient with this condition present on examination?

On examination, this patient has a port-wine stain in the first and second divisions of the trigeminal nerve. I would like to perform a skull X-ray looking for 'tramline calcification', examine the fundus for haemangioma of the choroids and ask about history of epilepsy.

These findings would be consistent with Sturge–Weber syndrome.

How is this condition inherited?

This is not an inherited condition.

What are the other complications of this condition?

In this condition there are capillary haemangiomas. The complications are:

- Eyes
  - glaucoma
  - optic atrophy
  - large eye (bupthalmos)
  - strabismus
  - choroid angioma
- Neurological
  - hemiparesis
  - hemianopia
  - low IQ
  - epilepsy

Treatment

- Antiepileptic drugs for fits
- Ophthalmology and neurology referral
- Supportive: special needs support, support groups, laser therapy for port wine stains

Case 8

Information for the candidate

You are: the medical doctor in the diabetic clinic.
Patient details: Mr Anthony Smith, aged 54 years.
This patient with type II diabetes was referred by the GP with the recent appearance of a ring-shaped skin lesion on the back of his hands. Latest bloods are as follows:

- HbA1c 6.9
- Cholesterol 4.5

- Sodium 143
- Potassium 4.2
- Urea 5.4
- Creatinine 92
- Full blood count normal
- Urine microalbumin normal

Your task: to assess the patient's problems and to identify what the skin lesion might be. You should address any questions raised by the patient.

Information for the patient

You are: Mr Anthony Smith, aged 54 years.
Your problem: rash on the back of your hands.
You have been referred by your GP because you have a rash on the back of your hands. If asked, this is not painful or itchy. It has been growing slowly for 2 months. Your doctor tried an antifungal cream for a few weeks. This had no effect. There have been no triggers for this skin rash, you feel well in yourself. The GP has now referred you to clinic as he thinks it could have something to do with your diabetes.

You have had type II diabetes for 5 years, and 3 years ago your GP told you that you had slightly elevated BP. You take metformin 500 mg twice daily and perindopril 4 mg once daily. If asked, all your checks including retinopathy, feet and urine are all up to date and have been normal. There is no other significant medical history. You are a non-smoker.
You should ask: what the rash is, what its significance is and what tests need doing.

Clinical consultation

In the 8 minutes you have, the candidate should:

- Take a detailed history about the skin rash – including time course, distribution, treatments used, pain/itching
- Enquire about the diabetes – including treatments used, complications, diabetic checks
- Enquire about compliance with medication and social history
- Examination – the emphasis of this should be on the skin lesion. Offer to perform fundoscopy, dipstick the urine and perform a foot check
- Discuss your diagnosis with the patient and the natural history of this condition

Discussion with the examiner

In the 2 minutes to discuss the case, the candidate might be asked:

Describe what you see

These are rings of smooth papules, which occur commonly on the back of the hands and fingers.

The patient has granuloma annulare.

What is the natural history of the condition?

This is usually a self-remitting condition. Treatment is not usually required.

What conditions is this associated with?

- Idiopathic
- Diabetes mellitus

What are the skin manifestations of diabetes?

- Due to insulin injecting – infection, lipoatrophy
- Necrobiosis lipoidica
- Granuloma annulare
- Diabetic foot ulcers
- Skin infections – bacterial, viral, fungal and yeast
- Lipodystrophy
- Diabetic dermopathy
- Eruptive xanthomas
- Diabetic bullae

Case 9

Information for the candidate

Your role: you are the medical doctor in casualty.
Patient details: Mrs Theresa Matthews, aged 45 years.
This lady presented with breathlessness.

The GP's letter mentions that she has deteriorated over the past 2 weeks, despite a course of amoxicillin. Over the past 6 months she has also complained of progressively worsening back pain.

The casualty doctors saw Mrs Matthews initially. She is now stable when you go to see her.

Her saturations were 94% on arrival but this has now picked up to 98% on 2 L O_2 via nasal cannula. Blood gases off air revealed a Po_2 of 9.0 kPa, otherwise normal. This has now improved with the oxygen.
Your task: to assess the patient's problems and answer any questions she raises.

Information for the patient

You are: Mrs Theresa Matthews, aged 45 years.
Your problem: breathlessness.
You have been admitted to casualty by your GP. Over the last 2 weeks, you have developed breathlessness. You visited the GP early into the illness and you were advised you had a chest infection. Antibiotics were prescribed but these were not effective. If asked, you have a slight dry cough and occasional wheeze. You experienced similar less intense episodes previously and were prescribed a salbutamol inhaler, which seemed to help.

You also have worsening back pain, which has been present for half a year. This has increased in intensity lately despite regular co-codamol. The pain is worse after rest and at night. It is improves when mobilizing. If asked, there are no problems with passing urine or faeces. There is no radiation of the pain and no numbness or tingling in the lower limbs. If asked, you have also noticed that your hands become excessively cold very easily. You have noticed your face looks different around the nose and lips.

You have no other significant medical history and are on no prescribed medications apart from those mentioned above. You are a lifelong non-smoker and work as a doctor's receptionist in a surgery. You should ask why you are now breathless and have back pain.

Clinical consultation

In the 8 minutes with the patient, the candidate should:

- Take a detailed history of the breathlessness
- Take a detailed history of the back pain, appreciating the difference between inflammatory and mechanical back pain
- Consider the possibility of a link between the breathlessness and back pain
- Perform a targeted examination, focusing particularly on inspection of the skin and hands, as well as examining the chest and back
- Explain to the patient what you think is wrong and what tests you propose.

Discussion with the examiner

In the 2 minutes to discuss the case, the candidate might be asked:

Describe your clinical findings

On examination, this patient is comfortable at rest. She has sclerodactyly of the fingers where the skin is smooth, shiny and tight. The pulp of the fingers is atrophied and there is calcinosis with subcutaneous calcium deposits. There are dilated nail-fold capillaries with loss of the distal part of the right middle finger and she appears to have Raynaud's phenomenon.

On examination of the face, the skin appears to be smooth, shiny and tight. She has a beaked nose and facial telangiectasia. There is perioral skin puckering with microstomia. Chest examination reveals fine end inspiratory crepitations. There is tenderness in the low back with a reduced range of movement.

These findings suggest a diagnosis of systemic sclerosis (Figure 7) complicated by pulmonary fibrosis and an inflammatory sounding lumbosacral back pain. I would like to complete my examination by performing a neurological examination of the lower limbs and checking the blood pressure to see if the patient has hypertension.

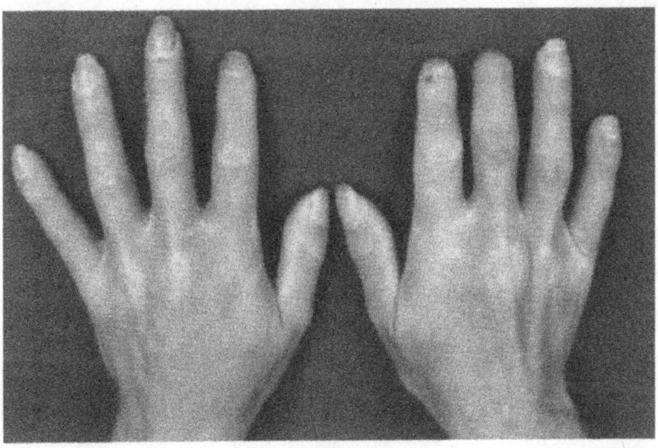

Figure 7 Scleroderma. Reproduced with permission of Aruna Dias from *Get Through MRCP Part 2: 350 Best of Fives*. London: RSM Press.

What is systemic sclerosis?

- This is a multiorgan connective tissue disorder characterized by fibrosis of the skin and other organs.
- It is more common in women.
- The cause is unknown but is likely to be multifactorial with genetic and environmental factors contributing to the development of the disease.

How do you classify the disease?

Systemic scleroderma

- Limited scleroderma or CREST syndrome, in which skin involvement is limited to the face, neck and distal limbs. Progression of the disease is slow. The CREST syndrome consists of:
  - **C**alcinosis
  - **R**aynaud's phenomenon
  - o**E**sophageal dysmotility
  - **S**clerodactyly
  - **T**elangiectasia.
- Diffuse scleroderma, in which skin involvement includes the trunk and proximal limbs. Internal organ disease is common and the disease is more severe than limited scleroderma.

Localized scleroderma

- Morphoea, in which there are plaques of sclerosis
- Linear sclerosis (coup de sabre) which presents on the frontal scalp

What are the other clinical features of systemic sclerosis?

Skin and nails

- Atrophic nails
- Ulceration especially of the fingertips
- Alopecia
- Vitiligo
- Oedema of the tissues

Gastrointestinal

- Dysphagia
- Reflux oesphagitis
- Small bacterial overgrowth (leads to steatorrhoea and malabsorption)
- Colonic diverticuli

Renal

- Malignant hypertension
- Renal failure

Cardiovascular

- Pericardial effusion
- Myocardial fibrosis

- Cardiomyopathy
- Conduction defects

Musculoskeletal

- Arthritis
- Myositis
- Myopathy

Respiratory

- Pleural effusions
- Pulmonary fibrosis
- Pulmonary hypertension
- Reflux pneumonitis
- Alveolar cell carcinoma can develop in areas of scarring

Other

- Dry eyes and dry mouth (Sjögren's syndrome)
- Other autoimmune disease

How would you investigate this patient?

Bloods

- Haemoglobin and haematinics, which may be reduced if there is malabsorption
- Renal function
- Antibodies
  - ANA positive in 90%
  - anti-centromere antibody is positive in limited systemic sclerosis
  - anti-Scl-70 antibody is positive in diffuse systemic sclerosis

Radiography of fingers

- X-ray of fingers for calcinosis
- X-ray of lumbosacral spine
- MRI lumbosacral spine to rule out other pathology, e.g. disc herniation, space-occupying lesion

Assessment for lung disease

- Lung function tests show restrictive pattern
- CXR and CT of the lungs may show pulmonary fibrosis (also need to rule out a PE or recurrent PEs for the worsening breathlessness)

Assessment for renal disease

- Urinalysis
- Consider renal biopsy

Assessment for gastrointestinal disease

- Barium studies
- Oesophageal manometry

Assessment of cardiac disease

- ECG to look for conduction defects
- Echocardiography to look at left ventricle and assess for fibrosis

How do you manage such patients?

General measures
- Education
- Physiotherapy to limit contractures
- Camouflage creams for areas of sclerosis

Telangiectasia
- Pulsed laser therapy

Raynaud's syndrome
- Gloves
- Hand warmers
- Calcium channel blockers
- ACE inhibitors
- Prostacyclin infusion
- Lumbar and digital sympathectomy

Gastro-oesophageal reflux disease (GORD)
- Proton pump inhibitors
- Pro-kinetic drugs

Malabsorption
- Nutritional supplements
- Antibiotics for gut bacterial overgrowth

Renal
- ACE inhibitors
- Calcium antagonists

Malignant hypertension
- ACE inhibitors

Pulmonary
- Prostacyclin infusions to treat pulmonary hypertension
- Steroids and immunosuppressant drugs such as cyclophosphamide, azathioprine and D-penicillamine for pulmonary fibrosis

Case 10

Information for the candidate

Your role: you are the elderly care doctor.
Patient details: Mrs Beatrice Jones, aged 85 years.
You are conducting a ward round on the elderly care ward. This patient was admitted to the ward 5 days ago having presented with acute confusion and frequency of urination. She was diagnosed with a urine infection. On admission she was tachycardic, febrile with a CRP of 100 mg/L and WCC of 15×10^9/L (neutrophilia). She responded well to intravenous co-amoxiclav. Earlier in the day her bloods revealed WCC of 10×10^9/L and CRP of 40×10^9/L. The observation chart shows that she has been afebrile for 48 hours; pulse rate and BP are normal.

The nurse looking after her mentions that she has complained of diarrhoea for the past 2 days.
Your task: to assess the patient's problems and address any queries she might have. You have not seen this lady before as you have just come off nights. You should also conduct a general review as part of a ward round.

Information for the patient

You are: Mrs Beatrice Jones, aged 85 years.
Your problem: admission for urinary infection and now diarrhoea.
You were admitted to the elderly care ward of your local hospital 5 days ago. The precise details of the admission are now a blur to you. You do, however, remember feeling unwell for the week leading up to this, with symptoms of burning when passing urine and visiting the toilet more frequently day and night. You also experienced sweating and feeling out of sorts.

Your daughter has since advised you that you started becoming confused during the week before admission. Examples she has given you are that you forgot family names, became unaware of where you were and forgot to cook dinner for friends you had invited over. On arrival, your friends noticed that something was not right so they called for an ambulance and you were admitted to the hospital. The confusion has now settled and you can answer the doctor's questions coherently.

Over the past 2 days you have developed loose watery stools, and are visiting the toilet every couple of hours. There is no blood, mucus or pus you have noticed. If asked, you have had no vomiting and no abdominal pain.

Prior to this illness you have never encountered problems with confusion. Your only medical history is hypertension and arthritis in the knees. Your regular medications include bendrofluazide and paracetamol. You cannot remember the doses.

You live alone and are fully independent. You have a daughter and son who live nearby and visit regularly.
You should ask: to be reminded of the reasons for admission and whether the episode of confusion is something to be worried about.

Clinical consultation

In the 8 minutes you have with the patient, the candidate should:

- Revisit the key reasons for her admission and enquire about how she has been during this admission
- Take a detailed history of the diarrhoea, enquire about food history/travel history and other unwell contacts on the ward
- Enquire about pre-morbid personality or any history of confusion
- Consider other causes of confusion, e.g. sepsis, medical history, drugs
- Establish baseline function (e.g. mobility, self-care, dressing) and social history
- Examine mental state with a mini-mental state examination and examine the abdomen
- Explain to the patient what you think about the diarrhoea and advise her of overall progress during this admission.

Discussion with the examiner

In the 2 minutes to discuss the case, the candidate might be asked:

What investigations, not already mentioned, would you wish to carry out into the acute confusion?

- Blood tests:
  - FBC
  - U&E
  - LFTs
  - bone profile
  - serum glucose
  - vitamin B_{12}/folate levels
  - TFTs
  - syphilis serology
- CXR to rule out chest infection
- ECG to rule out silent infarct
- Consider CT brain scan

How would you investigate this patient's diarrhoea?

- Stool culture for parasites/ova/cysts, as well as *C. difficile* toxin

How would you manage this patient?

- Discuss the case with the microbiologist with a view to stopping the IV augmentin (potential cause of the diarrhoea), as symptoms have settled and she has completed 5 days of treatment.
- Send off a repeat MSU specimen to confirm the UTI has resolved.
- Ensure that fluid balance is appropriate – consider IV fluid replacement.
- Adopt a multidisciplinary team approach, liaising with nursing staff and occupational therapists to determine how she will fare for discharge when medically fit. Involve the patient and family in this decision.

How would you manage this patient if the stool culture confirms *C. difficile*?

- Stop the augmentin.
- Liaise with the microbiologist about local guidelines – consider treating the *C. difficile* with oral metronidazole or vancomycin.
- Isolate the patient in a side room to prevent cross-infection.

Case 11

Information for the candidate

Your role: You are in clinic and about to see Mr Twist. The GP has sent you the following letter:

Patient details: Mr Twist, aged 35 years

Dear Cardiology

Thank you for seeing this 35-year-old gentleman, who came to see me as his wife complained that he was snoring. I have checked his blood pressure routinely and found it to be persistently high – 155/95 mmHg at best. I performed some baseline blood tests on him. Renal function is normal but he appears to be diabetic.

Could you please review him in view of his age and high blood pressure?

Yours sincerely

Dr Smith

Your task: To assess the patient's problems and try to work out why he has high blood pressure.

Information for the patient

You are: Mr. Twist, a 35-year-old man

Your problem: snoring. You saw your GP as your wife complained that your snoring has got worse. Your GP found that you have high BP and you then had a blood test, which showed that you were diabetic.

For several months, you have noticed that your peripheral vision is reduced but you have not got round to seeing the optician. You keep bumping into doors. You also noticed that your palms are more sweaty than normal. Your wedding ring has been very tight and you have had to take it off.

You recently attended a party with your old university friends and saw some old photographs. You think you look a bit different, with a large nose and lips. Your glove and shoe sizes have increased. The area under your armpits is now darker.

Your bowels are normal. You have no loss of sensation in your hands. There is no swelling in your neck. You have no other clinical features.

You should ask the doctor what is causing all these symptoms, what treatment options are available and the complications of this condition.

Clinical consultation

In the 8 minutes you have with the patient, the candidate should:

- Enquire about symptoms of acromegaly
- Examine the face, hands, axilla and visual fields. Note the presence of acromegalic facial features, acanthosis nigricans and a bilateral temporal field defect.
- Offer to measure the BP
- Advise the patient that he may have acromegaly
- Outline tests and treatment options.

Discussion with the examiner

In the 2 minutes to discuss the case, the candidate might be asked:

Describe your clinical findings

This 35-year-old man presented with high BP, reduced peripheral vision, sweaty palms and a change in facial appearance.

On examination, the patient has a large nose, lips and tongue with prominent supraorbital ridges. There is malocclusion of the teeth and an increase in the interdental spaces. The lower jaw is protruding (prognathism). The hands are large, sweaty, oily and spade shaped. The skin overlying them is thickened. There is no evidence of carpal tunnel syndrome or paraesthesia. There is a bitemporal peripheral visual field defect. Examination of the axilla reveals acanthosis nigricans.

These features suggest a diagnosis of acromegaly. I would like to complete my examination by checking his BP, perform a urine dipstick to check for glycosuria and examine the abdomen for hepatosplenomegaly.

How would you investigate this patient?

Blood tests

- GTT with GH response shows lack of suppression:
  - normally, GH levels are suppressed ≤ 2 mU/L after ingestion of 75 g of glucose
  - however, GH levels are not suppressed in acromegaly
  - GTT may also diagnose diabetes
- IGF-1 levels are raised
- Calcium levels – if raised, suggest MEN I syndrome

Assessment of anterior pituitary function

- The anterior pituitary gland produces other important hormones, in addition to GH, which may have been affected due to the pituitary adenoma.
- These hormones include TSH, ACTH and LH and FSH, which can all be directly measured or assessed via the insulin tolerance test.

Radiological tests

- MRI scan of the pituitary fossa detects the tumour
- CXR to determine presence of cardiomegaly
- Radiographs of hands and feet show terminal phalangeal 'tufting' and increased thickness of the heel pad

Other tests

- ECG
- Visual perimetry
- Comparison of old and new photographs to detect facial changes

How would you manage this patient?

Surgery

- Trans-sphenoidal hypophysectomy is the method of choice

Other options – if the surgery fails or the patient is unfit for surgery

- External irradiation
- Radioactive gold or yttrium implants
- Dopamine agonists such as bromocriptine and carbergoline
- Long-acting somatostatin analogues such as octreotide

What is acromegaly?

- Acromegaly is the abnormal enlargement of the skeleton and soft tissues caused by hypersecretion of GH after epiphysial fusion.
- It usually results from a pituitary macroadenoma.

What are the signs of active disease?

- Excessive sweating
- Glycosuria
- Hypertension
- Worsening visual field defect

What are the complications of acromegaly?

- Osteoarthritis
- Carpal tunnel syndrome
- Hypertension
- Hypercalciuria
- Hypertriglyceridaemia
- Renal stones
- Visual field defects
- Proximal myopathy
- Diabetes insipidus
- Chondrocalcinosis
- Diabetes mellitus
- Heart failure
- Hypercalcaemia
- Hypopituitarism
- Colonic tumours
- Hirsutism
- Obstructive sleep apnoea
- Hypogonadism causing amenorrhoea in women

What are the causes of macroglossia?

- Acromegaly
- Amyloidosis
- Down's syndrome
- Hypothyroidism

In what conditions can acanthosis nigricans occur?

- Acromegaly
- Obesity
- Type II diabetes mellitus
- Malignancy such as gastric carcinoma and lymphoma

What is MEN syndrome?

- There are two types of MEN.

Type I (Werner's syndrome)

- Autosomal dominant condition affecting the menin gene on chromosome 11
- Two or more of:
  - hyperparathyroidism
  - pituitary adenomas (prolactinomas or GH-secreting tumours in acromegaly)
  - pancreatic tumours (gastrinoma, insulinoma, glucagonoma)

Type IIa (Sipple's syndrome)

- Autosomal dominant disorder due to a defect in the *ret* gene on chromosome 10
- Two or more of:
  - hyperparathyroidism
  - phaeochromocytoma
  - medullary thyroid cancer

Type IIb

- Autosomal dominant disorder due to a defect in the *ret* gene on chromosome 10
- Characterized by mucosal neuromas, marfanoid habitus and two or more of:
  - hyperparathyroidism
  - phaeochromocytoma
  - medullary thyroid cancer

Case 12

Instructions for the candidate

Your role: You are the cardiology registrar in outpatient clinic
Patient details: Mrs Short, aged 25 years
You read the following GP letter.
Dear Cardiologist,
Thank you for seeing this 25-year-old lady. She recently joined a gym to lose weight and was found to have high blood pressure on her gym induction. She tells me she has put weight on and noticed more facial hair. I requested some blood tests to investigate for polycystic ovaries which revealed normal full blood count, renal function, liver function, thyroid function, sex hormone binding globulin and LH/FSH levels. She has also had an ultrasound scan which shows the ovaries are normal with no sign of polycystic ovaries.
I would be grateful for your opinion.
Yours sincerely,
Dr Smith
Your task: To assess the patient's problems and address any questions she raises.

Information for the patient

You are: Mrs. Short, aged 25 years
Your problem: high BP. You saw your GP because your gym instructor had noticed your BP was high. You have been trying to lose weight for some months now but seem to be putting it on despite dieting. You have noticed that you have more facial hair and your skin has more acne than ever before. You notice you have been bruising more easily. You also have some marks on your abdomen and are not sure what they are. You also noticed that your muscles in the thighs and arms seem a bit weaker than normal.

Your periods are irregular but not heavy. You have been feeling low but attribute this to problems in losing weight. You are not suicidal.

You want to know the cause of your symptoms, what treatment is available and whether this will help you lose weight.

Clinical consultation

In the 8 minutes with the patient, the candidate should:

- Enquire about the symptoms of Cushing's syndrome
- Examine the face and arms, noting the presence of purpura, abdominal striae and centripetal obesity
- Offer to measure the BP
- Advise the patient that she may have Cushing's syndrome
- Outline tests and treatment options.

Discussion with the examiner

In the 2 minutes to discuss the case, the candidate might be asked:

Describe your clinical findings

This lady presents with a history of weight gain, hirsutism and high blood pressure over the last few months. She has had irregular periods and she tells me her mood is low, but she is not suicidal. She has noticed some changes in the skin on her arms and abdomen.

This patient has centripetal obesity with slim legs and a buffalo hump. The face is round and plethoric. The skin shows both acne and hirsutism. Her skin is thin, and there are several purpuric patches on the arms, which are bruises. There are purple striae on the abdomen and proximal muscle weakness.

The likely diagnosis is Cushing's syndrome. I would like to complete my examination by checking the blood pressure and performing a urine dipstick to check for glycosuria.

How would you investigate this patient for Cushing's syndrome?

Establish hypercortisolaemia

- High midnight cortisol
- High 24-hour urinary free cortisol
- Low-dose dexamethasone suppression test

Establish the cause

- ACTH levels
- High-dose dexamethasone suppression test (Figure 8)

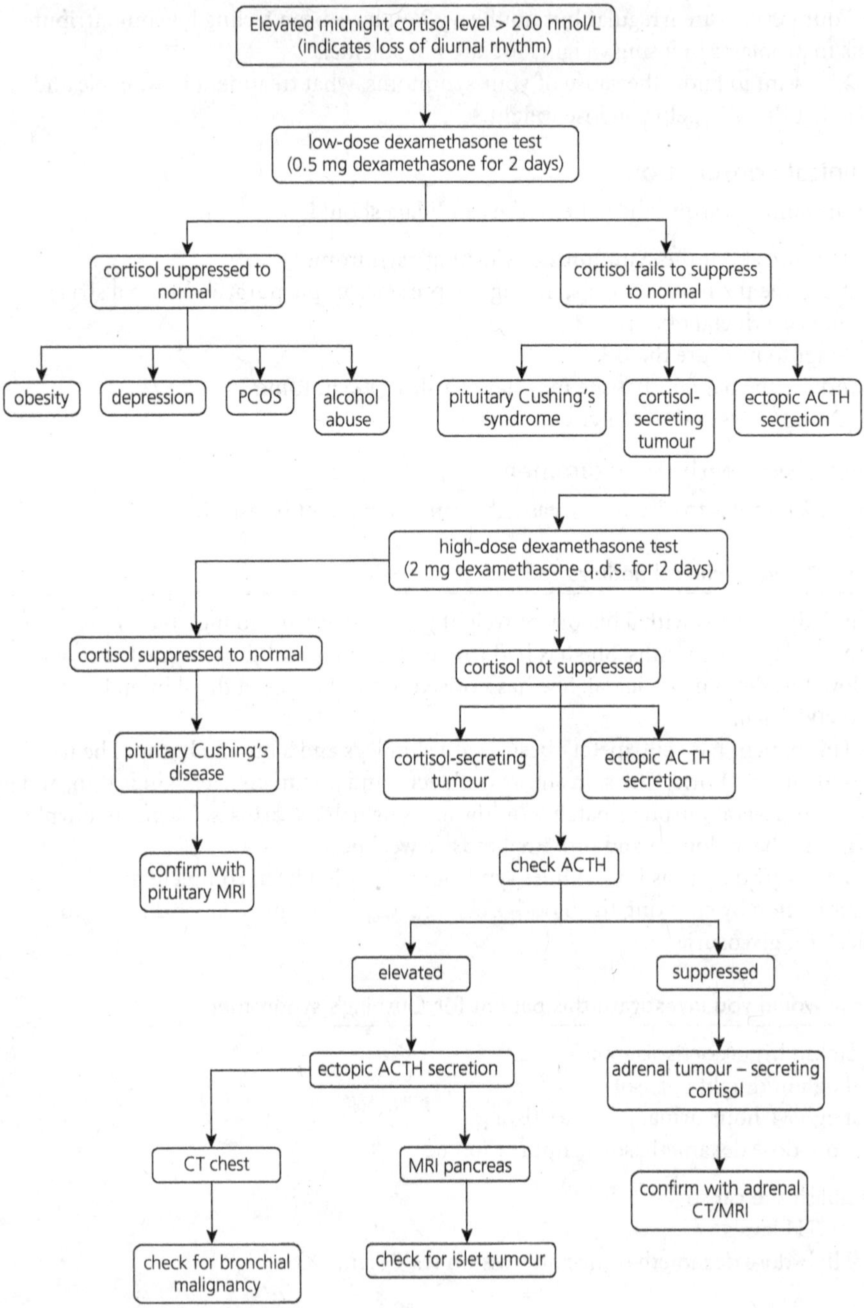

Figure 8 Diagnosis of Cushing's disease.

How do you manage patients with Cushing's disease?

- First-line treatment is with trans-sphenoidal hypophesectomy.
- Anti-adrenocortical drugs such as metyrapone or ketoconazole can be used pre-operatively or as an adjunct to surgical treatment.
- Radiotherapy if surgery is not successful or the patient is unfit for surgery.
- Bilateral adrenalectomy is used less commonly but may be needed occasionally.

What is Cushing's syndrome and what is Cushing's disease?

- Cushing's syndrome refers to the clinical features that result from persistent and inappropriately raised levels of glucocorticoid.
- Cushing's disease describes the specific condition in which an excessive amount of glucocorticoid is produced as a result of a pituitary tumour that secretes ACTH.

What are the causes of Cushing's syndrome?

- Prolonged exogenous use of steroids, e.g. for COPD or rheumatoid arthritis
- Pituitary adenoma secreting ACTH (Cushing's disease)
- Adrenal adenoma
- Adrenal carcinoma
- Ectopic ACTH secretion, e.g. small cell bronchial carcinoma, carcinoid tumour

What are the other features of Cushing's syndrome?

- Fatigue
- Sweating
- Osteoporosis
- Hypertension
- Impotence
- Depression
- Psychoses
- Supraclavicular fat pads
- Telangiectasia
- Diabetes mellitus
- Hyperpigmentation
- Infertility
- Anxiety
- Menstrual irregularities

What is Nelson's syndrome?

- This syndrome affects patients who have undergone bilateral adrenalectomy to treat Cushing's disease (i.e. they have an ACTH-secreting pituitary tumour).
- The loss of the adrenal glands leads to a massive surge in ACTH and MSH levels due to a lack of feedback inhibition, leading to hyperpigmentation and enlargement of the tumour which can cause mass effects, affecting the visual fields.
- It may be prevented by external radiation prior to or at the time of adrenalectomy.
- The syndrome is now rare as adrenalectomy is no longer a primary treatment for Cushing's disease.

What is Addison's disease?

This disease occurs as a result of autoimmune destruction of the adrenal gland, which leads to a deficiency of glucocorticoid and mineralocorticoid.

What symptoms do patients with Addison's disease present with?

- Hyperpigmentation of the skin
- Muscle weakness
- Diarrhoea and vomiting
- Sparse axillary and pubic hair
- Hypotension
- Symptoms and signs of other autoimmune conditions such as vitiligo
- Fatigue
- Weight loss
- Abdominal pain
- Depression

What is the cause of hyperpigmentation?

- Low levels of cortisol lead to a lack of feedback inhibition on the pituitary.
- This leads to a raised ACTH and melanocyte-stimulating hormone (MSH), leading to hyperpigmentation.

What other conditions are associated with Addison's disease?

- Vitiligo
- Hashimoto's thyroiditis
- Primary ovarian failure
- Graves' disease
- Pernicious anaemia

How would you investigate a patient for Addison's disease?

Blood tests
- Low sodium levels
- High potassium levels
- Hypoglycaemia
- Autoantibodies
- High ACTH levels

Other tests
- Early morning cortisol
- Short Synacthen test to confirm hypoadrenalism
- Long Synacthen test to differentiate between primary and secondary causes of hypoadrenalism

Imaging tests
- CXR to exclude malignancy or tuberculosis
- Abdominal radiograph to assess for adrenal calcification
- CT scan of the adrenal glands

How would you manage such a patient acutely (Addisonian crisis)?

- Rehydration with 0.9% saline and 5% dextrose if hypoglycaemic
- IV hydrocortisone
- Introduce fludrocortisone orally later
- Treat the underlying cause

How would you manage such a patient in the long term?

- Medic alert bracelet and steroid card
- Hydrocortisone and fludrocortisone orally
- Educate the patient about the need for steroids and advise increasing the dose if unwell

Name some other causes of hypoadrenalism

- Tuberculosis
- HIV
- Bilateral adrenalectomy (for cancer or as treatment for Cushing's syndrome)
- Amyloidosis
- Metastatic cancer
- Haemochromatosis
- Granulomatous disease
- Congenital adrenal hyperplasia
- Waterhouse–Friederichsen syndrome (meningococcal septicaemia leads to adrenal infarction)

What are the other causes of skin pigmentation?

- Cushing's disease
- Malabsorption syndromes
- Uraemia
- Nelson's syndrome
- Drugs such as amiodarone and minocycline
- Malignancy
- Cirrhosis
- Haemochromatosis
- Porphyria cutanea tarda

What is congenital adrenal hyperplasia?

- It is an autosomal recessively inherited group of disorders in which enzyme deficiencies lead to a deficiency of glucocorticoids ± mineralocorticoids.
- This leads to hyperstimulation of the adrenal gland by raised levels of ACTH from the pituitary gland, which results in excess production of testosterone and its precursors.
- This causes precocious puberty in males and virilization in females.

What is hirsutism?

- This is excessive hair growth in an androgen-dependent pattern in females.
- Women may have excessive hair growth in the beard area, around the nipples and in a male pattern on the abdomen.
- It is caused by:
  - increased androgen production
  - increased sensitivity of hair follicles to androgens.
- Androgens induce the transformation of fine vellus hair (small, straight and fair) into coarse terminal hair (larger, curlier, darker and more visible).

In contrast, hypertrichosis is the growth of hair on any part of the body, in excess of the amount usually present in persons of the same age, race and sex (excess androgen is not the source).

What conditions are associated with hirsutism?

Table 12 Conditions associated with hirsutism

Adrenal causes	Cushing's disease Virilizing tumours Congenital adrenal hyperplasia
Pituitary	Acromegaly Hyperprolactinaemia
Ovarian	Polycystic ovary syndrome Virilizing tumours
Drugs	Androgenic drugs Phenytoin

What treatments are there for hirsutism?

The underlying cause should always be treated if possible.

Table 13 Treatments for hirsutism

Physical methods	Waxing Shaving Plucking Threading Bleaching Depilation Electrolysis Laser treatment
Medical treatments	Anti-androgens such as cyproterone acetate – competitively inhibits androgens at peripheral receptors; can be used in a combined preparation called Dianette which also provides oral contraception
	Oestrogens or combined oral contraceptive pill – suppress ovarian androgen production in patients in whom the androgen is of ovarian origin
	Spironolactone – occupies androgen-binding sites on target tissues; has direct anti-androgenic properties
	Flutamide – androgen antagonist; unlike spironolactone, flutamide blocks androgen receptors without any glucocorticoid, progestational, androgenic or oestrogenic activity
	Finasteride – blocks 5α-reductase action and the peripheral conversion of testosterone to dihydrotestosterone
	Topical eflornithine cream – used to treat facial hirsutism; acts by irreversibly inhibiting ornithine decarboxylase

What are the autoimmune polyglandular syndromes?

Type I – two of:

- Addison's disease
- Hypoparathyroidism
- Chronic mucocutaneous candidiasis

Type II – two of:
- Addison's disease
- Autoimmune thyroid disease
- Type I diabetes mellitus

What is Schimdt's syndrome?

- This is the combination of Addison's disease and hypoparathyroidism.

Case 13

Instructions for the candidate

Your role: you are in Dermatology outpatients
Patient details: Mr Jones, aged 67 years
The GP has sent you the following letter:
Dear Dermatology
Thank you for seeing this 67-year-old gentleman who has a strange rash on his hands which has been present for some weeks.
Yours sincerely
Dr Smith
Your task: Establish the diagnosis and respond to the patient's questions

Information for the patient

You are: Mr Jones, aged 67 years
Your problem: you have developed a strange purplish rash on your knuckles a few weeks ago. If asked about other symptoms, you reveal that you are finding it difficult to get out of a chair or walk up the stairs. Your muscles feel tender, and generally you feel weaker in the upper arms and thighs. If asked, you reveal you have been a heavy smoker (30 to 40 cigarettes a day) for the last 40 years or so. You have noticed some generalized cough for the last few weeks but not had any change in your weight. You have no change in your bowels.
You should ask: you specifically want to know what has caused the rash, and why you feel weak.

Clinical consultation

In the 8 minutes with the patient, the candidate should:

- Enquire about the rash
- Enquire about symptoms of polymyositis
- Examine the hands, chest, upper and lower limbs
- Advise the patient that he may have dermatomyositis
- Explain that there is a link with malignancy – in this case the patient is a smoker so lung malignancy needs to be excluded
- Outline tests and treatment options.

Discussion with the examiner

In the 2 minutes to discuss the case, the candidate might be asked:

Describe your clinical findings

This gentleman presented with a rash on his knuckles. He has been a smoker of 30–40 cigerettes per day for many years and has a chronic cough but no weight loss. He tells me that he has muscle tenderness and weakness and finds it difficult to climb stairs.

There is a heliotrope rash around the eyes and Gottron's papules on the back of the hands. Nail-fold telangiectasia is present. Mr Jones has proximal muscle tenderness and weakness, and his reflexes are absent.

This is consistent with dermatomyositis (Figure 9). In view of the history of cough and heavy smoking, I would like to investigate this patient to exclude an associated lung malignancy.

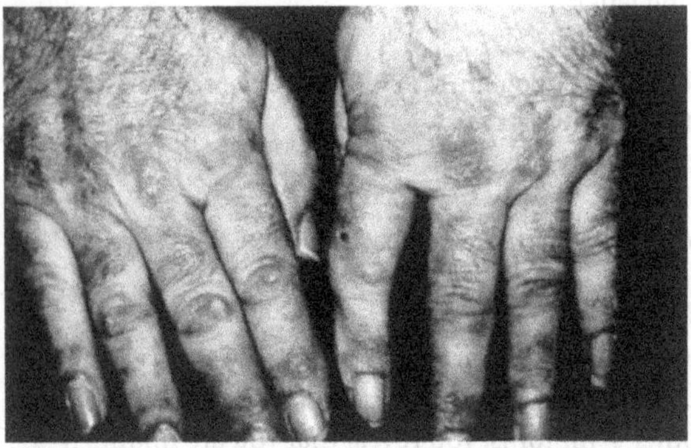

Figure 9 Dermatomyositis. Reproduced with permission of Aruna Dias from *Get Through MRCP Part 2: 350 Best of Fives*. London: RSM Press.

How would you investigate this patient?

Bloods

- CK levels are increased
- Myositis-specific antibodies:
  - anti-synthetase
  - anti-signal recognition particle (anti-SRP)
  - anti-Mi-2: chromodomain helicase DNA binding protein α

EMG

- Shows reduced duration and amplitude of action potentials, spontaneous fibrillation and increased polyphasic action potentials

Muscle biopsy

- Shows muscle necrosis, phagocytosis of muscle fibres, and an inflammatory infiltrate

Tests to investigate underlying malignancy

- FBC to check for anaemia
- LFTs and calcium to check for metastatic spread of disease
- CXR to look for lung mass. If present, proceed to CT scan and bronchoscopy and biopsy

What are the diagnostic criteria?

- Polymyositis:
  - proximal, symmetrical muscle weakness
  - elevation of serum muscle enzymes
  - characteristic EMG abnormalities
  - muscle biopsy showing myositis
- Dermatomyositis:
  - as above with skin changes

What are treatment options?

- Treat the underlying cause (removal of tumour or treatment of associated connective tissue disease).
- Oral steroids are the main form of treatment. Prednisolone is started initially at 20–60 mg per day and then reduced to maintenance therapy.
- Immunosuppressive therapy with second-line agents such as methotrexate and azathioprine may be required.
- IV immunoglobulin is used for refractory cases.

Discuss the complications of this condition

- Polymyositis is an inflammatory disease of the muscle which becomes known as dermatomyositis when there is the characteristic rash described above.
- Complications include:
  - proximal muscle weakness
  - dysphagia due to oesophageal involvement
  - calcium deposits in subcutaneous tissue and skin
  - vasculitis affecting the skin and viscera
  - malignancy: most commonly bronchial, breast and stomach
  - respiratory: aspiration pneumonia, respiratory failure
  - cardiac: CCF, arrhythmias
  - association with connective tissue disorders.

What is the prognosis for dermatomyositis?

Both dermatomyositis and polymyositis have a 5-year survival of over 80% if treated early.

Case 14

Information for the candidate

Your role: you are the medical SHO covering ward referrals
Patient details: Mr Bone, aged 67 years

You have been contacted by the orthopaedic team to review a man on the ward who has been admitted for a knee operation. This is their referral letter in the notes.

Dear Medics

Thank you for seeing this 67-year-old gentleman who has had a left knee replacement. He is recovering on the ward. He has a history of diabetes and is on metformin 500 mg three times a day, simvastatin 20 mg o.d. and ramipril 20 mg o.d. His blood pressure is normal at 127/79 mmHg. However, his HbA_{1c} is high at 8.7%. Other bloods, including cholesterol, are normal.

Please could you review him, in view of his high HbA_{1c}, for further treatment and have a look at his eyes as he is still complaining of blurred vision.

Many thanks

Orthopaedic Team

Information for the patient

Your are: Mr. Bone, aged 67 years

Your problem: poor diabetic control and blurred vision. You saw your optician a few months ago as your eyesight was getting worse. You are short sighted and wear glasses to read. Your optician advised you to see your GP for a blood test to check for diabetes as there were some changes in your eyes.

You saw your GP and were started on metformin 500 mg three times a day and advised to lose weight. You have found this difficult as you have arthritis of your knees, cannot walk far and needed a knee replacement. You take all your tablets daily. You are hoping to lose weight when you have had your knee replacement. Your GP started you on tablets to control your blood pressure and cholesterol.

You have been admitted to have your knee operated on and are waiting to be discharged. The orthopaedic team have told you your diabetes is not controlled well enough, and you may need other tablets. You mentioned your eyesight still is poor. If asked, you do not smoke and have never had any problems with chest pain, stroke, TIAs or kidney disease.

You should ask: you specifically want to now why you need more tablets, why your vision is blurred and how it can be managed.

Clinical consultation

In the 8 minutes with the patient, the candidate should:

- Enquire about the history of diabetes (how long ago it was diagnosed, symptoms and treatment)
- Enquire about compliance with his medications
- Enquire about eye symptoms
- Perform fundoscopy and diagnose proliferative retinopathy
- Explain the findings to the patient
- Advise a referral to the ophthalmology department for possible photocoagulation
- Explain the importance of BP and cholesterol control
- Explain the importance of diabetic control and the need to add in gliclazide
- Advise the patient to see his GP in 2 months to recheck HbA1c to check if gliclazide has improved diabetes control.

Discussion with the examiner

In the 2 minutes to discuss the case, the candidate might be asked:

Describe your clinical findings

This is a 67-year-old diabetic gentleman who has had a left knee replacement. He is on treatment with metformin, ramipril and simvastatin. His BP and cholesterol are normal but he has a high HbA_{1c} at 8.7%. He is short sighted but has noticed that his vision is becoming more blurred.

Fundoscopy reveals diabetic retinopathy (describe stage and treatment options).

In addition, I would start the patient on gliclazide to improve his diabetes control. I would advise this gentleman about weight loss, consider orlistat and ask him to be followed up by his GP.

What are the features of diabetic eye disease?

In the examination, any of the following stages of diabetic eye disease can present. The features are described below. You should be familiar with all of them. In addition, you should be very familiar with the NICE guidelines for the management of type I and type II diabetes.

Background diabetic retinopathy

On examination, there are:

- microaneurysms
- dot and blot haemorrhages
- hard exudates.

These findings suggest that the diagnosis is *background diabetic retinopathy* (Figure 10).

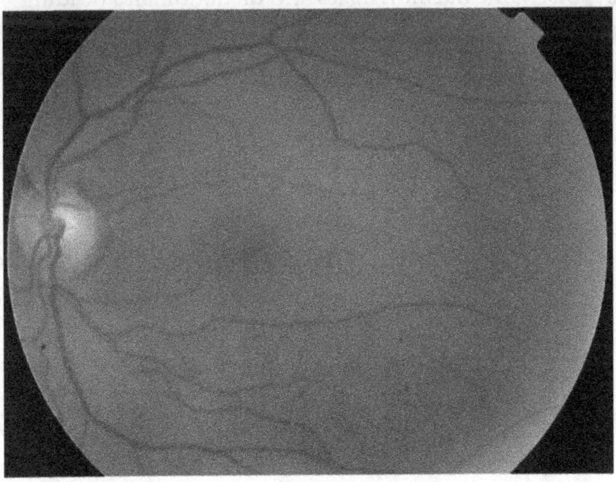

Figure 10 Background diabetic retinopathy. Reproduced with permission of Hiten G. Sheth.

Pre-proliferative diabetic retinopathy

On examination, there are microaneurysms, dot and blot haemorrhages and hard exudates. There are also:

- cotton wool spots
- flame haemorrhages
- dilatation and beading of retinal veins.

These findings suggest that the diagnosis is *pre-proliferative diabetic retinopathy* (Figure 11).

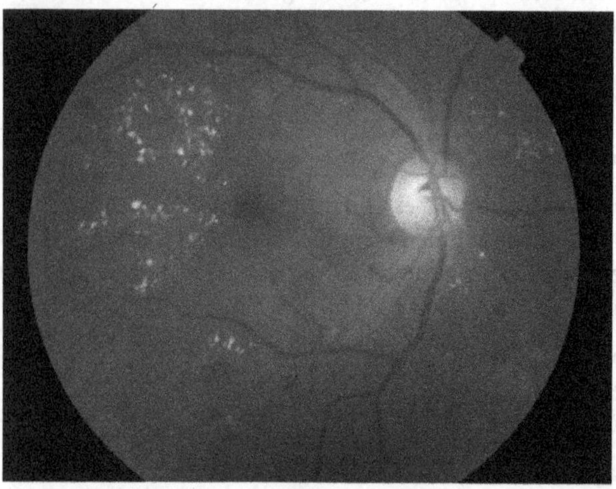

Figure 11 Pre-proliferative diabetic retinopathy. Reproduced with permission of Shamira Perera.

Proliferative diabetic retinopathy

On examination, I can see microaneurysms, blot haemorrhages and hard exudates. There are also cotton wool spots, flame haemorrhages and dilatation and beading of retinal veins. I can also see:

- Multiple new vessels at the disc
- Multiple new vessels elsewhere
- Photocoagulation scars

These findings suggest that the patient has *proliferative diabetic retinopathy* (Figure 12) treated by photocoagulation (see Figure 13).

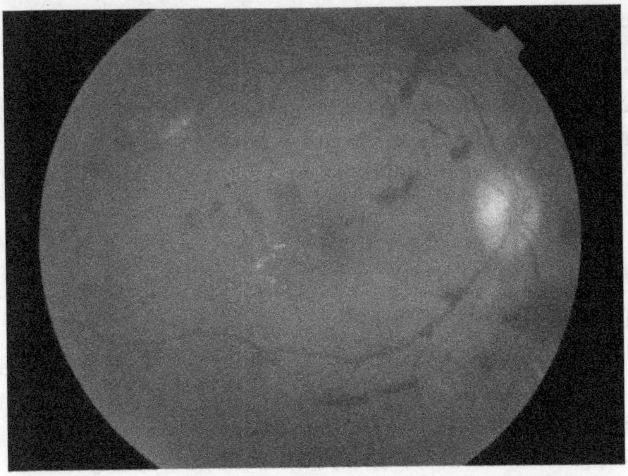

Figure 12 Proliferative retinopathy and diabetic maculopathy. Reproduced with permission of Shamira Perera.

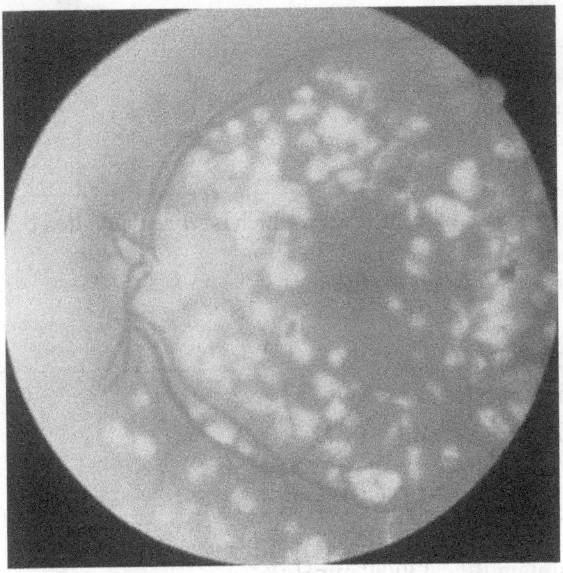

Figure 13 Photocoagulation scars. Reproduced with permission of Aruna Dias from *Get Through MRCP Part 2: 350 Best of Fives*. London: RSM Press.

Advanced diabetic eye disease

On examination, there are features of diabetic eye disease (state which of the above signs) with:

- Vitreous haemorrhages and scars
- Retinal detachment
- Cataracts
- Rubeosis iridis (abnormal blood vessels on the surface of the iris)

These findings suggest the patient has *advanced diabetic eye disease.*

Diabetic maculopathy

On examination, there are features of diabetic eye disease (state which of the above signs). In addition there is a circinate formation of hard exudates (suggesting oedema) near the macula in the right eye. I would like to check for impaired central vision.

What do you know about diabetic eye disease?

- It is the commonest cause of blindness in the UK.
- The risk of developing diabetic retinopathy increases with the duration of having diabetes.
- Good diabetic control slows the development of retinopathy.
- After 20 years of having type I diabetes, nearly all patients have some degree of retinopathy. Type I diabetics tend to develop proliferative retinopathy.
- After 20 years of having type II diabetes, 80% of patients have some degree of retinopathy. Type II diabetics tend to develop maculopathy.

What are microaneurysms?

- These are bulges in weak vessel walls.
- They appear as red dots on the fundus.

What are exudates?

- These occur as a result of lipid leaking from vessels, which has been engulfed by macrophages.
- They appear as yellow–white deposits on the fundus.

What are cotton wool spots?

- These are ischaemic or infarcted areas of the retina.
- They appear as white, fluffy spots.

How do you manage patients with diabetic eye disease?

- Maintain good glycaemic control – aim for HbA_{1c} to be below 7.5%.
- Treat hypertension and maintain BP < 130/80 mmHg.
- Annual screening with digital retinal photography.
- Consider photocoagulation.
- Encourage the patient to stop smoking.

When should you refer a patient with diabetes to an ophthalmologist?

- Background retinopathy: routine referral
- Pre-proliferative retinopathy: routine referral
- Proliferative retinopathy: urgent referral
- Maculopathy: routine referral

In what circumstances does sudden deterioration occur?

- Pregnancy
- Hypertension
- Anaemia
- Renal failure
- Poor diabetic control

What are the indications for photocoagulation?

- Pre-proliferative retinopathy
- Proliferative retinopathy
- Maculopathy

Tell me about photocoagulation

- Focal photocoagulation targets specific vessels at risk of bleeding.
- Pan-retinal photocoagulation prevents the ischaemic retinal cells secreting angiogenesis factors and causing revascularization.
- When directed against areas of macular oedema, photocoagulation reduces leakage and improves reabsorption of retinal oedema.
- It reduces the risk of severe visual loss.

What ocular complications may develop with diabetes?

- Cataracts
- Ocular nerve palsies (especially CN VI palsy)
- Central retinal artery occlusion
- Central vein occlusion
- Rubeosis iridis
- Rubeotic glaucoma
- Increase risk of infection (conjunctivitis and herpes zoster)

How do you grade hypertensive eye disease?

Table 14 Hypertensive eye disease

Grade I	Silver wiring (due to thickened arteriolar walls)
Grade II	Arteriovenous nipping (narrowing of the veins as arterioles cross them)
Grade III	Cotton wool spots (areas of infarction) and flame haemorrhages
Grade IV	Papilloedema

- Hard exudates (leakage of lipid from vessels) causing a 'macular star' can also occur.

What are the causes of hypertension?

- Essential hypertension
- Renal disease such as renal artery stenosis, GN and polycystic kidney disease
- Coarctation of the aorta
- Endocrine disorders such as Cushing's disease, Conn's syndrome, or phaeochromocytoma

How would you investigate a patient with high blood pressure?

- Bloods, including:
  - renal function
  - fasting glucose
  - lipids
- Urine for protein and casts
- Electrocardiography
- CXR
- Further investigations may be necessary:
  - autoimmune screen
  - urinary catecholamines
  - USS of the kidneys
  - renal biopsy

Case 15

Instructions for the candidate

Your role: you have been asked to see a ward referral by your registrar
Patient details: Mr Freeman, aged 79 years
You have been handed the following referral letter:
Dear Medics
This gentleman was admitted 3 weeks ago for an elective hip replacement for osteoarthritis. He had a difficult post-operative period, and ended up in ICU for management of heart failure. He did well after a few days and has returned on to the ward for recovery and rehabilitation. On our ward round today, the house officer noted that his pupils were unequal. Mr Freeman says that his pupils have always been equal, and we are not sure why this has happened.
His medications include paracetamol 1 g q.d.s. for residual hip pain, aspirin 75 mg o.d., furosemide 40 mg o.d., ramipril 2.5 mg o.d., bisoprolol 1.25 mg o.d., simvastatin 20 mg o.d. and omeprazole 20 mg o.d.
The cardiologists have reviewed him and optimized him from a heart failure point of view. Please review him specifically with regards to his unequal pupils.
Many thanks
Orthopaedic Team

Information for the patient

You are: Mr Freeman, aged 79 years
Your problem: Unequal pupils
You were admitted for an elective hip replacement to manage your hip pain due to severe osteoarthritis. After the operation, you became short of breath and ended up in ICU. You are not sure exactly what happened but apparently your heart was not working as well as it should have done.

When you left ICU, you came back to the ward and have started to mobilize. The pain in your hip is much better and you only require paracetamol for the pain. You were seen by the cardiology team and your medications were changed around. You do not know what they are all called.

On the ward round this morning, one of the doctors noted your pupils were unequal. The left one seems smaller than the right. However, your vision is as good as ever. You do not have diabetes.

You should ask: the doctor why your pupils are unequal in size.

Clinical consultation

In the 8 minutes with the patient, the candidate should cover the following:

- Enquire about the patient's hospital stay
- Perform an ophthalmologic examination
- Examine for causes of Horner's syndrome
- Advise the patient that he has Horner's syndrome.

Discussion with the examiner

In the 2 minutes to discuss the case, the candidate might be asked:

Describe your clinical findings

This 79-year-old man was admitted for an elective hip replacement 3 weeks ago. He had hip pain due to severe osteoarthritis. Post-operatively he developed heart failure and was managed in ICU. He is currently mobilizing and requires only paracetamol for pain relief. His heart failure has been reviewed by the cardiology team. However, on the ward round, one of the doctors noted that his pupils were unequal in size.

On examination, the left pupil is meiotic (due to paralysis of the pupil dilator muscle). There is ipsilateral ptosis (due to paralysis of Muller's muscle), enophthalmos and anhydrosis. There is a fresh scar in the supraclavicular area which may have been due to central line insertion while in ICU. There is no cervical lymphadenopathy or wasting of the small muscles of the hands.

The diagnosis is Horner's syndrome following central line insertion.

Examination tips

- Examine the supraclavicular area for scars or enlarged lymph nodes.
- Examine the neck for carotid aneurysms and tracheal deviation (Pancoast tumour).
- Examine the hands for small muscle wasting, loss of ulnar sensation, clubbing of the fingers (seen in Pancoast's tumour or syringomyelia).
- Examine for cerebellar signs and optic disc atrophy seen with multiple sclerosis.

What are the causes of Horner's syndrome?

- It is caused by any lesion in the sympathetic nervous system as it travels from the sympathetic nucleus, through the brainstem and spinal cord to the level of C8/T1/T2, to the sympathetic chain and plexus.
- Lesions are classified as first-, second- or third-order neuron disorders.
- Congenital Horner's syndrome is associated with heterochromia of the iris.

First-order neuron disorders

- Brainstem strokes (lateral medullary syndrome)
- Brainstem demyelination (e.g. multiple sclerosis)
- Syringomyelia and syringobulbia
- Pontine haemorrhage
- Basal skull tumours
- Basal meningitis

Second-order neuron disorders (pre-ganglionic or central lesions)

- Pancoast's tumour
- Mediastinal tumour
- Cervical lymphadenopathy
- Cervical rib
- Thyroid enlargement
- Neck surgery or trauma

Third-order neuron disorders

- Carotid dissection
- Carotid and aortic aneurysms

What are the features of Horner's syndrome?

Table 15 Features of Horner's syndrome

Miosis	due to paralysis of the papillary dilator muscle
Ptosis	due to paralysis of the upper tarsal muscle
Enophthalmos	due to paralysis of the muscle of Muller
Reduced sweating	due to a central lesion with loss of sweating to half of the head, arm and upper trunk

Case 16

Information for the candidate

Your role: you are the doctor covering the outpatient clinic
Patient details: Mrs Scott, aged 67 years
This lady has been referred to you by her GP with the following letter:
Dear Gastroenterology
Thank you for reviewing this 67-year-old lady who tells me she has been suffering from constipation over the last 2 or 3 months. She has not lost weight or had any bleeding per rectum. On examination, there is no abdominal mass. Her FBC/renal function tests/LFTs are normal, as were three faecal occult blood samples. She has tried lactulose and senna, which helped slightly, but I would be grateful if you could review her as she is not keen on continuing with laxatives long term.
Yours sincerely
Dr Peacock

Information for the patient

You are: Mrs Scott, aged 67 years
Your problem: constipation
You have been suffering from constipation for 3 months. You open your bowels every 3 days or so which is a struggle. There is no abdominal pain, bleeding per rectum, melaena or jaundice. You have no diarrhoea. You have not lost weight. Actually, you have been getting heavier, and are upset that, despite exercising at the gym over the last 6 months, you have noticed you have gained weight.

If asked, you have noted that you feel quite cold, frequently needing a few layers to keep you warm. You have also found that you are more tired than normal, and struggle with the gym. You have not noticed any change in voice. You take laxatives only, which help, but you do not want to take these long term. If asked, your sister and mother have hypothyroidism. You noticed your neck is bigger than normal, but you have attributed this to gaining weight overall.

You should ask: you specifically want to know what is causing your constipation and how it can be resolved.

Clinical consultation

In the 8 minutes with the patient, the candidate should cover the following:

- Enquire about the symptoms of constipation and exclude a gastrointestinal cause
- Ask about features of hypothyroidism
- Ask about other autoimmune disorders
- Ask about medication and family history
- Examine the hands, pulse, eyes, neck, heart and reflexes
- Advise the patient that she may have hypothyroidism
- Outline tests and treatment options.

Discussion with the examiner

In the 2 minutes to discuss the case, the candidate might be asked:

Describe your clinical findings

This 67-year-old woman has a 3-month history of constipation. She has no other gastrointestinal symptoms such as intermittent diarrhoea, abdominal pain, jaundice, bleeding per rectum or melaena. She has noticed weight gain and intolerance to cold and has been more tired than normal.

On general examination, she is overweight. She has coarse facial features with peri-orbital oedema and facial puffiness. There is loss of the outer third of the eyebrows. The skin is dry and cold. The voice is hoarse and husky. Her pulse is slow at 60 beats/minute, and her ankle jerk reflexes are delayed. She appears to have proximal myopathy because she has difficulty getting out of a chair, but does not have cerebellar signs. There is a smooth goitre present but no bruit, cervical lymphadenopathy or retrosternal extension.

The likely diagnosis is hypothyroidism.

Additional points

- The presence of a goitre suggests Hashimoto's disease.
- The presence of exophthalmos would suggest the patient has Graves' disease and has become hypothyroid following treatment with radioactive iodine or thyroidectomy.
- When examining a goitre, comment on:
  - presence of multinodular goitre/solitary nodule in the thyroid/diffusely enlarged goitre
  - whether there is retrosternal extension of the goitre

- presence or absence of cervical lymphadenopathy (suggests malignancy) or bruit
- whether the patient is euthyroid/hyperthyroid/hypothyroid on the basis of the presence or absence of sweaty palms, tremor of the hands, pulse rate, reflexes and lid lag

What blood tests may you perform on a patient that you suspect is hypothyroid?

- FBC – may show anaemia with macrocytosis
- TSH – elevated in thyroid failure and reduced in pituitary failure
- Free thyroxine – may be reduced
- Thyroid autoantibodies
- Cholesterol – may be raised
- CK and LDH – may be raised

How would you investigate patients with a goitre?

Ultrasound

- Determines size and number of nodules
- Determines whether cystic or solid

Fine needle aspiration biopsy

- Helps to provide a histological diagnosis

Nuclear scans

- Toxic adenomas are hot
- Malignant nodules and thyroiditis are cold

How would you manage patients with hypothyroidism?

- Oral levothyroxine daily for life
- Titrate dose according to TSH levels and clinical symptoms
- Titrate dose up slowly in elderly as treatment with thyroxine can unmask angina

What are the causes of hypothyroidism?

Primary

- Autoimmune Hashimoto's thyroiditis
- Post-thyroidectomy
- De Quervain's thyroiditis
- Post-partum thyroiditis
- Iodine deficiency
- Congenital causes
- Drugs such as radioactive iodine, amiodarone or lithium

Secondary

- Pituitary failure
- Hypothalamic failure

What symptoms may patients with hypothyroidism present with?

Cardiovascular

- Anaemia with macrocytosis
- Bradycardia
- Hypertension

Neurological

- Delayed reflexes
- Cerebellar syndrome
- Peripheral neuropathy

- Hypercholesterolaemia
- Cardiac failure
- Coronary artery disease
- Pericarditis
- Carpal tunnel syndrome
- Proximal myopathy
- Dementia
- Depression

Other

- Weight gain
- Tiredness
- Hypothermia
- Intolerance of cold
- Constipation
- Menorrhagia
- Infertility

What other diseases are associated with hypothyroidism?

- Grave's disease
- Pernicious anaemia
- Vitiligo
- Addison's disease
- Diabetes mellitus
- Rheumatoid arthritis
- Sjögren's syndrome

What causes the puffy skin changes in hypothyroid patients?

Accumulation of hyaluronic acid and water content of the tissue leads to a thickened, puffy appearance of the skin.

What is the differential diagnosis of a single thyroid nodule?

- Palpable nodule in a multinodular goitre
- Thyroid adenoma
- Thyroid cyst
- Thyroid carcinoma

What is the differential diagnosis of a diffusely enlarged thyroid?

- Simple goitre
- Graves' disease (treated if patient is euthyroid)
- Hashimoto's thyroiditis
- De Quervain's thyroiditis
- Secondary to goitrogens such as lithium
- Congenital enzyme defects such as Pendred's syndrome

What symptoms may a patient with a thyroid lump present with?

- Stridor
- Dysphagia
- Dysphonia
- Hoarse voice suggests pressure on the recurrent laryngeal nerve (usually due to malignancy)

What types of thyroid cancer do you know about?

Papillary carcinoma

- 80% of thyroid cancers
- Good prognosis
- Spreads to cervical lymph nodes – distant spread is rare
- Usually able to be removed through surgery
- Radioiodine can be used post-operatively to ablate residual cells followed by TSH suppression with thyroxine

Follicular carcinoma

- Affects the middle aged
- Spreads haematogenously to bones and lung
- Usually able to be removed through surgery
- Radioiodine can be used post-operatively to ablate residual cells followed by TSH suppression with thyroxine

Anaplastic carcinoma

- Affects the elderly
- Carries a poor prognosis
- Highly malignant and spreads to the trachea and oesophagus

Medullary carcinoma

- Rare
- Spreads locally to the lymph nodes and also to the bones and lungs
- Arises from the para-follicular or C-cells of the thyroid and secretes calcitonin
- Can arise sporadically or be transmitted in an autosomal dominant pattern as part of the MEN II syndrome

Lymphoma

- Usually occurs in patients with Hashimoto's disease
- Treatment is with radiation

Case 17

Information for the candidate

Your role: you are the medical SHO on call in A&E
Patient details: Miss Anna Smith, aged 28 years
Your next patient presents with palpitations. Her initial ECG shows a sinus tachycardia of 120 beats/minute. While waiting to be reviewed, her heart rate has settled. A repeat shows a sinus rhythm of 90 beats/minute. Her bloods reveal normal FBC, renal and liver function.
Your task: to find the cause of the palpitations and answer the patient's questions about management

Information for the patient

You are: Miss Anna Smith, aged 28 years
Your problem: palpitations. You have had this problem for 2 weeks.

The palpitations occur sporadically throughout the day. There is no specific triggering factor. The episodes last approximately 20–30 minutes and subside spontaneously. You usually sit down and stop what you are doing when the palpitations start. You feel as if your heart is beating very quickly.

You attended A&E today as the palpitations lasted longer than normal. They settled after about 45 minutes today, while you were in A&E. If asked, you have no chest pain or shortness of breath. If asked, you notice that you seem to be hot most of the time over the last few months. You have been particularly sweaty, even in normal temperature environments. You have lost 3–4 kg despite eating more than before. You still have periods, but they have become lighter over the last three cycles. They are still regular in pattern and you do not have period pains. Your bowels are normal. You have not noticed any tremor of the hands and your vision is normal. If asked, you think your neck may look a bit bigger than normal.

You were adopted at birth and are not sure of any family history. You are not on any medications, do not use illicit drugs or smoke. You drink a glass of wine on special occasions only and have one of two cups of tea or coffee daily.

You should ask: the doctor what is causing all these symptoms, what treatment options are available and what are the complications of this condition.

Clinical consultation

In the 8 minutes with the patient, the candidate should cover the following:

- Enquire about the onset of the palpitations
- Ask about cardiac symptoms such as chest pain and shortness of breath
- Ask about symptoms of hyperthyroidism
- Ask about medication and family history
- Ask about alcohol and caffeine intake
- Examine the hands, pulse, eyes, neck and reflexes
- Advise the patient that she may have hyperthyroidism
- Outline tests and treatment options

Discussion with the examiner

In the 2 minutes to discuss the case, the candidate might be asked:

Describe your clinical findings

This 28-year-old woman presents to the A&E department with a 2-week history of palpitations. Her ECG initially showed a sinus tachycardia which settled after some time in A&E. She has no cardiac features but does have symptoms of hyperthyroidism with palpitations, intolerance to heat, weight loss despite eating well and lighter periods than normal. She does not have any visual symptoms.

On examination, she has sweaty palms, thyroid acropachy and a fine tremor of the hands when outstretched. She has a normal pulse of 90 beats/minute, with a regular rhythm. She has a small diffuse goitre with a bruit. On examination of the eyes, she has exophthalmos, chemosis, ophthalmoplegia and diplopia (see Figure 14 for an example of thyroid eye disease). She also has lid lag and lid retraction. She has brisk reflexes. She has purplish, elevated, symmetrical lesions on her shins which suggest pre-tibial myxoedema.

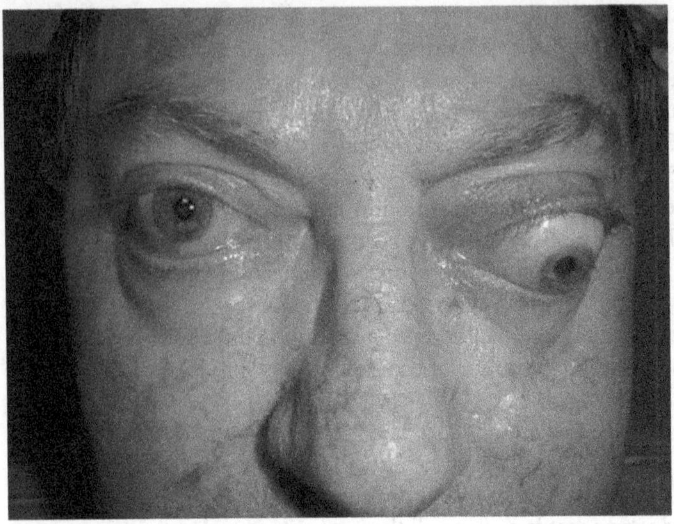

Figure 14 Thyroid eye disease. Reproduced with permission of Shamira Perera.

Discussion with the examiner

In the 2 minutes to discuss the case, the candidate might be asked:

What symptoms can patients with hyperthyroidism present with?

- Weight loss
- Increased appetite
- Heat intolerance
- Excessive sweating
- Palpitations
- Shortness of breath
- Diarrhoea
- Oligomenorrhoea
- Insomnia
- Fatigue
- Irritability and nervousness
- Muscle weakness

How would you investigate this patient?

ECG (if not already performed)

- Look for AF or other cardiac cause of palpitations

Blood tests

- FBC
- TFTs
- Thyroid autoantibodies

Radioisotope scanning

- Increased uptake of iodine in Graves' disease
- Reduced iodine uptake in thyroiditis and thyroid malignancy

How would you manage this patient?

Anti-thyroid drugs

- Carbimazole or propylthiouracil can be used.
- These drugs may take several weeks to control thyroid levels.

- β-blockers such as propanolol can be used in the interim for symptom control.
- There are two treatment regimens when using anti-thyroid drugs:
  - **block and replace regimen** in which a high-dose anti-thyroid drug is used and levothyroxine added when the patient becomes euthyroid
  - **reducing dose regimen** in which the anti-thyroid drug is started at high dose and titrated down as the patient becomes euthyroid
- The anti-thyroid drugs are continued for 18–24 months and then stopped to assess the success of the treatment.
- Approximately 50% of patients will relapse. These patients can be managed by:
  - repeat anti-thyroid drugs
  - radioiodine
  - subtotal thyroidectomy

Radioiodine

- Patients treated with radioiodine should not be in close contact with other people for 12 days and avoid non-essential contact with pregnant women and children for 30 days.
- Hypothyroidism following treatment is a common side effect. These patients are treated with replacement levothyroxine.
- Contraindications include:
  - breastfeeding
  - pregnancy
  - iodine allergy
  - active eye disease
  - patients who cannot avoid close contact with others

Surgery

- Indications include:
  - large goitre
  - patient preference
  - non-compliance with drugs
  - relapse of hyperthyroidism after treatment with anti-thyroid drugs

What is exophthalmos caused by?

- This is due to infiltration of lymphocytes and mucopolysaccharide into the orbital fat and intraorbital muscles.
- It can occur when the patient is hyperthyroid or euthyroid and can persist or worsen despite treatment of hyperthyroidism.

What are the complications of thyroid eye disease?

- Chemosis
- Exposure keratitis
- Corneal ulceration
- Ophthalmoplegia and diplopia

How do you manage exophthalmos?

Mild and moderate disease

- Advise the patient to stop smoking
- Methylcellulose eye drops and lubricating eye ointment
- Protective glasses, which may be tinted to protect eyes
- Prism glasses or surgery on the extraocular muscles to treat diplopia

Severe disease

- High-dose steroids
- Orbital irradiation
- Plasma exchange
- Surgical decompression

What are the causes of hyperthyroidism?

Primary

- Graves' disease
- Toxic adenoma
- Multinodular goitre
- Post-partum thyroiditis
- De Quervain's thyroiditis
- Excess thyroxine replacement

Secondary

- TSH-secreting pituitary adenoma
- Excessive release of TRH from hypothalamus
- Hydatidiform mole
- Choriocarcinoma
- Struma ovarii

What is Graves' disease?

- This is an autoimmune condition in which TSH receptor IgG antibodies bind to the TSH receptor and stimulate it, causing hyperthyroidism.
- It is the commonest cause of hyperthyroidism.
- Females are affected more than males (5 : 1).

In a patient with hyperthyroidism, what specific signs suggest Grave's disease?

- Exophthalmos
- Thyroid acropachy
- Pre-tibial myxoedema

What do you know about post-partum thyroiditis?

- It is a self-limiting disease which presents up to 12 months post partum.
- It presents with a painless goitre or hyperthyroidism.
- It has a hyperthyroid phase in which thyroid destruction causes increased release of thyroxine. This is followed by a phase of hypothyroidism as stores are depleted.
- Radioiodine uptake is low in the hyperthyroid phase.
- Thyroid peroxidase antibodies are present.

What do you know about De Quervain's thyroiditis?

- It is a painful thyroiditis due to a viral illness. Patients are often febrile.
- It has a hyperthyroid phase in which thyroid destruction causes increased release of thyroxine. This is followed by a phase of hypothyroidism as stores are depleted.

- Radioiodine uptake is low in the hyperthyroid phase.
- ESR is raised.

What is struma ovarii?

- This is an ovarian teratoma with thyroid tissue.

What are the complications of hyperthyroidism?

- AF
- Hypertension
- Cardiac failure
- Proximal myopathy
- Hair loss
- Onycholysis
- Palmar erythema
- Osteoporosis

Case 18

Information for the candidate

Your role: your consultant has asked you to see the following ward referral
Patient details: Mrs Hawthorne, aged 77 years
The orthopaedic team have written the following referral:
Dear Medics
This lady was admitted 2 weeks ago for an elective knee replacement for osteoarthritis. Her knee is in fabulous condition and healing well. However, she is having difficulty mobilizing and is complaining of stiffness around the hip. Movements of the hip joint are normal and radiographs show only mild osteoarthritis. Her bloods reveal normal FBC, renal and liver function.
We are puzzled by her symptoms and would be grateful for your review.
Many thanks
Orthopaedic Team

Information for the patient

You are: Mrs Hawthorne, aged 77 years
Your problem: Difficulty walking
You were admitted for an elective left knee replacement. You had severe pain in your knee due to arthritis and needed many painkillers. Following the operation, your pain is settling, and the orthopaedic team have told you that the knee looks fine.

You are receiving physiotherapy to help with your mobility before you go home but do not seem to be doing as well as you would like. You live alone in a flat on the first floor so it is important that you can walk properly. You feel very stiff around the hip and shoulder, which are painful, but you are not weaker per se. The stiffness is worse in the morning and worsened since being in hospital. You feel very tired but are not sure why. If asked, you have had some temporal headaches while on the ward. Recently, when brushing your hair, you have noticed that your scalp is tender

on the left side. If asked, you have not noticed any problems when chewing or eating. If asked, your vision is normal.
You should ask: the doctor what is causing all these symptoms, what treatment options are available and the complications of this condition.

Clinical consultation

In the 8 minutes with the patient, the candidate should cover the following:

- Enquire about the symptoms of stiffness
- Ask about symptoms related to temporal arteritis
- Examine the upper and lower limbs
- Examining the scalp for temporal artery thickening
- Offer fundoscopy
- Offer to check the BP in both arms to exclude aortic arch involvement
- Advise the patient that she may have polymyalgia rheumatica and temporal arteritis
- Outline tests and treatment options

Discussion with the examiner

In the 2 minutes to discuss the case, the candidate might be asked:

Describe your clinical findings

This 77-year-old woman was admitted for an elective left knee replacement in view of severe pain from osteoarthritis. Her knee is healing well. She has had pain and tenderness around the hip and shoulders for some weeks, but this has worsened since her hospital admission. It is worse in the morning. Radiographs of the hip and shoulders are normal.

In addition, she has been feeling tired and describes temporal headaches and scalp tenderness. She has no visual symptoms or jaw claudication.

On examination, she has bilateral muscle tenderness around the shoulders and pelvic girdle muscles. There is no wasting of muscles. She has a good range of movement at the shoulder and hip, but movements are painful. She has tenderness over the temporal artery but no thickening of the vessel. Her vision is normal.

These features suggest a diagnosis of polymyalgia rheumatica and temporal arteritis.

What is polymyalgia rheumatica (PMR)?

- PMR is a condition of unknown aetiology that is characterized by symmetrical pain and stiffness involving the proximal muscle groups – the pectoral and pelvic girdles.
- The condition is most common in women over the age of 50 years.
- There is an association with temporal arteritis.

What symptoms occur in this condition?

- There is pain and stiffness at the shoulders, upper arms, neck, and hips.
- Symptoms are worse first thing in the morning.

- True weakness does not occur although power and range of movement may be limited due to pain and stiffness.
- Patients have difficulty turning in bed, rising from a bed or chair, or raising arms above shoulder height.
- Systemic symptoms include tiredness, depression, night sweats, fever, loss of appetite and weight loss.
- Symptoms of temporal arteritis may also occur.

What investigations would you consider in this patient?

Bloods

- FBC may reveal a normochromic, normocytic anaemia.
- ESR is usually markedly elevated; it returns to normal with treatment.
- CRP is usually elevated.
- ALP may be raised – this returns to normal with treatment.
- Liver transaminase levels are normal.
- Autoimmune screen is normal.
- CK and calcium levels are normal.

How would you treat patients with PMR?

- Oral corticosteroid treatment with prednisolone
- Start with 15–20 mg o.d. and slowly reduce over 1 month to 10 mg daily
- Taper dose thereafter by 1 mg every 4–6 weeks
- Steroid-sparing drugs such as methotrexate and azathioprine can be used in patients who require a longer duration of steroids
- Patients may need steroid therapy for 2 years, therefore calcium, vitamin D and bisphosphonates should be considered to prevent the complications of osteoporosis. A proton pump inhibitor may be considered for gastric protection

What is temporal arteritis?

- This is a vasculitis affecting medium-size and large arteries.
- It almost exclusively affects individuals over 50 years, and is more common in women than men.
- Although any large artery may be affected, the branches of the carotid artery result in the majority of the symptoms and signs. The condition primarily affects the aorta and its extracranial branches. Intracranial arteries are only rarely involved.
- PMR precedes or accompanies giant cell arteritis in more than 50% of cases.

What are the clinical features of temporal arteritis?

- Malaise
- Fever
- Anorexia and weight loss
- Temporal headache
- Scalp tenderness
- Jaw claudication

- Transient visual disturbances
- Symptoms of polymyalgia rheumatica

What are the signs of temporal arteritis?

- Temporal arteries may be tender, dilated, inflamed, thickened or cord-like.
- The artery may be pulsatile and bruits may occur if there is partial occlusion.

What are the complications of temporal arteritis?

- Scalp ulceration
- Ischaemic optic neuropathy causing sudden loss of vision
- Central retinal artery occlusion (less common)
- Angina and myocardial infarction
- Aortic arch syndrome
- Thoracic aorta aneurysm or dissection
- Intracerebral artery involvement (rare) can cause hemiplegia and epilepsy

How do you diagnose temporal arteritis?

The American College of Rheumatology considers that three of the five diagnostic criteria must be met to support a diagnosis of temporal arteritis.

Table 16 Diagnostic criteria for temporal arteritis

Criterion	Definition
Patient older than 50 years at disease onset	Development of symptoms or findings beginning when a patient is older than 50 years
New headache	New-onset or new type of localized pain in the head
Temporal artery abnormality	Temporal artery tenderness on palpation or decreased temporal artery pulse, unrelated to arteriosclerosis of the cervical arteries
Elevated ESR	ESR greater than 50 mm/hour
Abnormal biopsy	Vasculitis characterized by a mononuclear cell infiltration or granulomatous inflammation, usually with multinucleated giant cells

How do you manage patients with temporal arteritis?

Ophthalmology referral

Visual disturbance is an ophthalmological emergency and requires immediate referral to ophthalmology.

Steroid therapy

- Oral prednisolone 40–60 mg per day if no visual symptoms
- Oral prednisolone 60–80 mg per day if visual symptoms present
- Intravenous methylprednisolone may be necessary in cases of impending vision loss
- Treatment should continue even if there is loss of vision in one eye as aggressive treatment will prevent visual loss in the contralateral eye, which has a 20–50% chance of becoming affected in a short period of time

- Steroid treatment is gradually tapered by 5–10 mg every 2 weeks until reaching 20 mg per day and then more slowly. The effectiveness of treatment is monitored through the patient's ESR
- Aspirin 75 mg daily (if no contraindications)
- Proton pump inhibitor for gastroprotection
- Calcium, vitamin D and bisphosphonates for bone protection

Other points

- Monitor FBG regularly in view of high-dose steroids.
- Maintain a high index of suspicion for infections during courses of high-dose steroid treatment as this may mask symptoms and signs of infection.

Case 19

Information for the candidate

Your role: you are the medical SHD in the Rheumatology outpatient clinic

Patient details: Mrs Nowak, aged 58 years

The GP sent you the following letter:

Dear Rheumatology

Thank you for seeing this 58-year-old Polish lady who recently joined our practice. She moved to the UK 4 years ago and has only just registered with a general practice. She came to see me because she was feeling tired. She has a history of rheumatoid arthritis for which she takes diclofenac when needed. When she lived in Poland she was apparently on some form of medication for her rheumatoid arthritis but she cannot remember what it was or how often she took it. I performed some baseline blood tests which showed she had a normochromic, normocytic anaemia with a haemoglobin of 9.5 g/dL. Liver and renal function are normal. She is struggling with her hands in terms of function and I am concerned about her haemoglobin level, and wonder if she is anaemic because of NSAID treatment.

I would be grateful for your review.

Yours sincerely

Dr Smith

Information for the patient

You are: Mrs Nowak, aged 58 years

Your problem: worsening hand pain with known rheumatoid arthritis. You moved to the UK 4 years ago. If asked why, you reveal that you felt employment opportunities were better in the UK. You began working for a cleaning company but stopped because the pain in your hands was getting worse. You were told you have rheumatoid arthritis 10 years ago in Poland and were started on some tablets but you cannot remember what they were called or how often you took them. You stopped taking these tablets as you could not afford them in Poland. You have not taken any medication for your rheumatoid arthritis except for diclofenac that you get from the walk-in centre. They advised you to register with a GP because the pain in your hands was getting worse. You recently registered with a GP and when you saw him you also told him how tired you were feeling. You subsequently had a blood test but do not know the result. You do not have any symptoms of gastric reflux or peptic ulcer disease. You have no melaena or haematemesis.

If asked about family history, you explain that your sister, who still lives in Poland, has rheumatoid arthritis which is rather disabling, as did your mother, who passed away several years ago.

You should ask: you specifically want to know about the blood test, what it means and the options for treating your rheumatoid arthritis.

Clinical consultation

In the 8 minutes with the patient, the candidate should cover the following:

- Enquire about the history of rheumatoid arthritis (how long ago it was diagnosed, treatment and symptoms)
- Ask about NSAID usage and peptic ulcer symptoms such as dyspepsia, epigastric pain, haematemesis and melaena
- Ask about symptoms of anaemia such as shortness of breath and feeling tired
- Explain that the blood test shows a low haemoglobin level. Explain that this accounts for the patient's tiredness
- Examine the hands and assess function
- Advise that treatment options include steroids and DMARDs
- Offer to start the patient on methotrexate
- Explains that this drug is administered weekly and her FBC will need to be monitored
- Explain that she will also need to take folic acid
- Explain that treatment will reduce the progression of the disease
- Explain that other investigations such as a CXR would be useful to check her lungs and spirometry would assess her lung function prior to starting on methotrexate
- Offer referral to occupational therapy to provide aids to help, for example, with opening cans
- Offer a follow-up appointment

Discussion with the examiner

In the 2 minutes to discuss the case, the candidate might be asked:

Discuss your clinical findings

On examination, this woman has rheumatoid arthritis of the hands (Figure 15). She has a symmetrical deforming arthropathy affecting the proximal IPJs and the MCPJs. The terminal IPJs are spared. There is wasting of the small muscles of the hand and ulnar deviation of the fingers. There is a 'swan neck' deformity and Boutonniere's deformity of the fingers. She has nodules at the elbows.

When assessing function, she has difficulty fastening buttons and turning keys. She has pallor of the conjunctiva suggesting anaemia. I would need to investigate the cause of anaemia further but, as it is a normochromic, normocytic anaemia, it is likely to be due to anaemia of chronic disease.

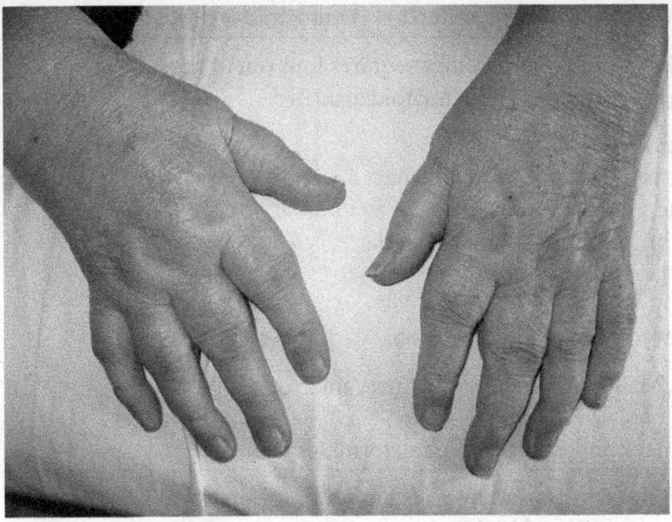

Figure 15 Rheumatoid arthritis. Reproduced with permission of Mr Wai Weng Yoon.

How would you investigate this patient?

Bloods

- Haemoglobin to confirm anaemia (check MCV to decide if microcytic, normocytic or macrocytic)
- Check iron, vitamin B_{12} and folate levels
- ESR and CRP may be raised

Synovial fluid analysis

- Elevated white cell count
- Low glucose
- Low C3 and C4

Radiograph of joints involved

- Joint space narrowing
- Juxta-articular osteoporosis
- Joint erosions
- Cyst formation
- Joint destruction
- Subluxation

What is rheumatoid arthritis?

- This is a chronic, inflammatory, autoimmune disease mediated by the formation of IgG antibodies produced by plasma cells in the joint synovium.
- These IgG antibodies activate the complement mechanism leading to production of pro-inflammatory cytokines such as TNF-α which cause joint destruction.
- It affects 1% of the population with a female to male ratio of 3 : 1.
- The peak incidence is between 25 and 55 years.

What do you know about diagnostic criteria in rheumatoid arthritis?

- The American College of Rheumatology requires four out of the following criteria to be present to diagnose rheumatoid arthritis:

1. Morning stiffness > 1 hour for > 6 weeks
2. Swelling of at least three types of joints for > 6 weeks*
3. Swelling of hand joints for > 6 weeks
4. Symmetrical joint involvement for > 6 weeks
5. Nodules
6. RF positive
7. Radiological features such as joint erosions

*Joints can be PIPJ, MCPJ, the wrist, elbow, knee, ankle or MTPJ.

Explain what swan neck and Boutonniere's deformities are

- Swan neck deformity results from hyperextension of the proximal IPJ with fixed flexion of the terminal IPJ and MCP joint.
- Boutonniere's deformity results from a flexion deformity of the proximal IPJ with extension contracture of the terminal IPJ and MCP joints.

What factors are associated with a poorer prognosis?

- Positive RF
- Many joints affected
- Extra-articular disease
- Joint erosions early in disease
- Severe disability at presentation
- High ESR or CRP at presentation

What are the causes of anaemia?

- Anaemia of chronic disease
- Microcytic anaemia due to gastrointestinal bleeding from NSAIDs
- Megaloblastic anaemia due to folic acid deficiency or associated pernicious anaemia
- Felty's syndrome
- Bone marrow suppression due to treatment with DMARDs such as gold, methotrexate, sulfasalazine, penicillamine

What are the other clinical features present?

Hands
- Palmar erythema
- Triggering of the fingers
- Z deformity of the thumb

Musculoskeletal

- Elbow, knee and foot involvement
- Cervical spine involvement, whereby atlantoaxial joint subluxation can lead to spin cord compression
- Bursitis
- Tenosynovitis

Respiratory

- Pleural effusions
- Pulmonary fibrosis
- Pulmonary nodules
- Caplan's syndrome
- Bronchiolitis obliterans

Neurology

- Peripheral neuropathy
- Mononeuritis multiplex
- Cervical myelopathy
- Carpal tunnel syndrome

Eyes

- Episcleritis
- Scleritis
- Cataracts
- Scleromalacia and scleromalacia perforans

Cardiovascular

- Pericarditis
- Myocarditis

Dermatology

- Nail-fold infarcts
- Pyoderma gangrenosum
- Leg ulceration
- Raynaud's phenomenon

Other

- Cushingoid features due to steroid therapy
- Secondary amyloidosis
- Other autoimmune disorders such as Sjögren's syndrome

How do you manage patients with rheumatoid arthritis?

Conservative management

- Education
- Exercise and physiotherapy
- Splinting to protect joints
- Occupational therapy

Drug management
- NSAIDs
- DMARDs
- Steroids
- Inhibitors of TNF-α action

Surgery
- Joint replacement
- Tendon transfer

What is the role and mechanism of action of NSAIDs in rheumatoid arthritis?

- NSAIDs help with pain, stiffness and swelling but do not control the underlying disease process.
- NSAIDs inhibit the enzyme COX and so reduce the synthesis of prostaglandins, which are responsible for causing inflammation.
- COX is present in two different forms: COX-1 and COX-2.
- COX-1 is essential for the maintenance of normal physiological states in many tissues including the kidney, gastrointestinal tract, and platelets. COX-1 activation in the gastric mucosa leads to production of the prostaglandin called prostacyclin, which helps protect the gastric tissues from insult. Hence, inhibition of COX-1 leads to gastrointestinal damage.
- COX-2 is less widely expressed but leads to production of prostaglandins that mediate inflammation.
- The anti-inflammatory effect of NSAIDs results from inhibition of COX-2.
- The COX-2 inhibitor drugs such as celecoxib inhibit COX-2 but not COX-1. They have fewer side effects such as gastrointestinal bleeding but increase the risk of thrombotic events such as stroke and myocardial infarction.

Name some common and important side effects of NSAIDs

Gastrointestinal
- Dyspepsia
- Peptic ulceration and haemorrhage

Renal
- Renal failure
- Interstitial nephritis

Other
- Exacerbation of asthma
- Erythema multiforme
- Hepatitis

Tell me about the role of DMARDs in rheumatoid arthritis. Name their mechanism of action and common side effects

- These drugs are used to delay disease progression and reduce the severity of the disease (Table 17).

Table 17 DMARDs: mode of action and common side effects

Drug	Indications	Mode of action	Side effects	Monitoring
Chloroquine and hydroxychloroquine	Rheumatoid arthritis SLE Malaria	Lysosyme stabilization	Retinal damage Rash	Fundoscopy and visual fields: baseline and every 6 months
Methotrexate	Rheumatoid arthritis Psoriasis Cancer chemotherapy	Competitive antagonist of dihydrofolate reductase	Diarrhoea and vomiting Hepatotoxicity Pneumonitis Rheumatoid nodules Bone marrow suppression	FBC, U&E, LFTs, CXR Baseline lung function tests
Sulfasalazine	Rheumatoid arthritis Ankylosing spondylitis Psoriatic arthritis	Active compound liberated in gut by action of gut flora	Rash Hepatitis Pancreatitis Oligospermia Bone marrow suppression	FBC, U&E, LFTs
Gold	Rheumatoid arthritis	Immunomodulatory drug	Rash Mouth ulcers Glomerulonephritis Proteinuria Bone marrow suppression	FBC, U&E, LFTs Urinalysis
Penicillamine	Rheumatoid arthritis Wilson's disease Copper and lead poisoning Cystinuria	Immunomodulatory drug Chelates metal ions	Rash Proteinuria Mouth ulcers Bone marrow suppression Autoimmune disease: SLE, myasthenia gravis, thyroiditis	FBC, U&E, LFTs Urinalysis

continued

Table 17 DMARDs: mode of action and common side effects *(Continued)*

Drug	Indications	Mode of action	Side effects	Monitoring
Azathioprine	Rheumatoid arthritis SLE Inflammatory bowel disease Myasthenia gravis	Inhibits DNA synthesis	Nausea and vomiting Jaundice Skin malignancy Bone marrow suppression	FBC, U&E, LFTs
Cyclophosphamide	Rheumatoid arthritis SLE Vasculitis Nephrotic syndrome Chemotherapy	Interferes with DNA synthesis	Bone marrow suppression Nausea and vomiting Interstitial nephritis Azoospermia Haemorrhagic cystitis	FBC Urinalysis
Ciclosporin	Rheumatoid arthritis SLE Eczema Psoriasis	Prevents T-cell activation	Nephropathy Hypertension Hirsutism Gum hypertrophy Lymphoma	FBC, U&E Urinalysis

What is the role of steroids?

- They can be given orally in acute flare-ups or as background therapy.
- Acute, painful joint swelling which does not resolve can be treated by intra-articular steroid therapy.
- Calcium supplements and bisphosphonates should be given to prevent the development of osteoporosis.

What are the side effects of steroids?

- Bruising
- Hirsutism
- Round face
- Hypertension
- Impaired glucose tolerance
- Peptic ulcer disease
- Weight gain
- Acne
- Cataract
- Glaucoma
- Osteoporosis
- Infections especially recurrent fungal infections

What do you know about the anti-TNF-α drugs?

Etanercept

- Indications include rheumatoid arthritis, ankylosing spondylitis and psoriatic arthritis.
- This is a fusion protein consisting of a recombinant TNF-α receptor and the Fc constant region of human IgG.
- It is administered through subcutaneous injection twice a week when other DMARDs have failed.
- It can be given with methotrexate or alone.
- It can cause reactivation of tuberculosis.

Infliximab

- Indications include rheumatoid arthritis, ankylosing spondylitis, psoriasis and Crohn's disease.
- Infliximab is a chimeric mouse anti-TNF monoclonal antibody that binds to and inhibits human TNF-α.
- It is administered intravenously when other DMARDs (including methotrexate) have failed.
- It is given at 0, 2 and 6 weeks and then every 8 weeks thereafter.
- It must be used in combination with methotrexate.
- It can cause reactivation of tuberculosis.

Case 20

Information for the candidate

Your role: you are making your way to the outpatient clinic when you receive a call about one of the patients you have just seen on the ward round
Patient details: Mr Singh, aged 57 years

This patient was admitted for treatment of pneumonia and has responded well to a course of IV antibiotics. He is due to be discharged tomorrow. You saw him on the ward round and wrote his discharge summary. The only medication he is to be discharged on is bendroflumethiazide 2.5 mg o.d.

The nurse looking after him bleeps you to review him. He has developed a painful, swollen left knee.

Your task: to assess the problem and explain your management to the patient

Information for the patient

You are: Mr. Singh, aged 57 years

Your problem: swollen left knee whilst in hospital

You were admitted to hospital for treatment of a severe chest infection. You have been in for 6 days so far and are due for discharge tomorrow. You have had some IV antibiotics and changed to oral tablets today. Unfortunately when you tried to walk to the toilet, you noticed your left knee was very swollen. You struggled to walk to the toilet because of the pain. You have never had any pain in your knees before.

If asked, you had a flare-up of your left big toe when on holiday in France 2 months ago. Your wife gave you some diclofenac, which she had with her because she uses it for back pain, which did help but it took a week to settle down. If asked, you drink about 3 pints of beer a day. You are not dependent on alcohol. If asked, your diet is rich in meat. You particularly enjoy red meat. You do not have occasional pain in the small joints of your hands and feet. You have no systemic systems. You were started on some tablets for high BP about 3 months ago. You are otherwise well.

You should ask: you want to know what has caused the knee swelling, what treatment is available and if you can still go home tomorrow, as planned.

Clinical consultation

In the 8 minutes with the patient, the candidate should:

- Enquire about the symptoms of knee pain and swelling
- Ask about systemic features such as fever, to exclude septic arthritis
- Ask about other joint pains
- Ask about alcohol intake and diet
- Examine the knee and hands and look for tophaceous deposits at the elbows and ear
- Advise the patient that he may have gout
- Advise the patient to reduce his alcohol intake and change his diet
- Suggest a change in medication for his BP as his current tablets can predispose to gout
- Outline tests and treatment options
- Reassure the patient that he can still be discharged tomorrow if he is happy mobilizing.

Discussion with the examiner

In the 2 minutes for discussion, the candidate might be asked:

Describe your clinical findings

This man has developed a painful swollen knee while an inpatient following successful treatment of pneumonia with IV antibiotics. He has a history of a painful left first MTPJ that resolved after treatment with diclofenac. He is on bendroflumethiazide 2.5 mg o.d. and drinks 3 pints of beer daily. He has a diet rich in meat.

On examination, this patient is afebrile. His left knee is swollen, red and hot. He has full range of movement at the knee and is able to weight bear. In addition, he has asymmetrical swelling of the small joints of the hands (and feet). He has tophi of the helix of the ear and olecranon bursa.

This patient appears to have tophaceous gout, with an acute attack affecting the knee. His risk factors include being overweight, having a diet rich in meat, drinking heavily and being on a thiazide diuretic.

What do you understand about gout?

- Gout is a disorder of purine metabolism which leads to increased levels of uric acid.
- This results in recurrent attacks of synovitis due to urate crystal deposition.
- It affects males more than females with a male to female ratio of 20 : 1.

What are the causes of raised urate levels?

Primary causes

- Idiopathic
- Lesch–Nyhan syndrome: HGPRT deficiency

Secondary

- Increased production of purines or uric acid:
  - myeloproliferative disorders
  - lymphoproliferative disorders
  - psoriasis
  - chemotherapy
  - severe exercise
- Increased ingestion of purines or uric acid:
  - diet high in purines (meat, alcohol)
- Reduced uric acid excretion:
  - renal failure
  - drugs such as thiazides, ciclosporin and aspirin

How would you investigate this patient?

Bloods

- Raised serum uric acid levels – but they can also be normal or reduced

Joint aspiration

- Negatively bi-refringent needle-shaped crystals

Joint radiographs
- Punched-out erosions distant from the joint margin
- Joint destruction

How would you treat this patient?

Acute attack
- NSAIDs
- Colchicine – but patients may not be able to tolerate it due to diarrhoea
- Oral steroids (short course) may be required

Prophylaxis
- Allopurinol (xanthine oxidase inhibitor) or probenecid
- Prophylaxis should not be commenced during an acute attack
- Indications for prophylaxis include:
  - > four attacks of gout per year
  - one attack of polyarticular gout
  - tophaceous gout
  - urate kidney stones

What is pseudogout?

- This is a clinical syndrome that is clinically similar to gout.
- However, the underlying cause is the deposition of calcium pyrophosphate crystals in the joints (rather than urate crystals).
- Treatment is with NSAIDs and intra-articular steroid injections in severe cases.
- There is no prophylaxis.

What are the causes of pseudogout?

- Hyperparathyroidism
- Hypomagnesaemia
- Haemochromatosis
- Ochronosis
- Hypothyroidism
- Hypophosphataemia
- Wilson's disease

How do you diagnose a patient with pseudogout?

- Joint aspiration shows positively bi-refringent brick shaped crystals.

PART II

REVISION MATERIAL

11

CHAPTER 1 SUPPLEMENTARY CASES

OPHTHALMOLOGY

1. Blue sclera

What are the causes of blue sclera (Figure 16)?

- Osteogenesis imperfecta
- Ehlers–Danlos syndrome
- Pseudoxanthoma elasticum
- Marfan's syndrome

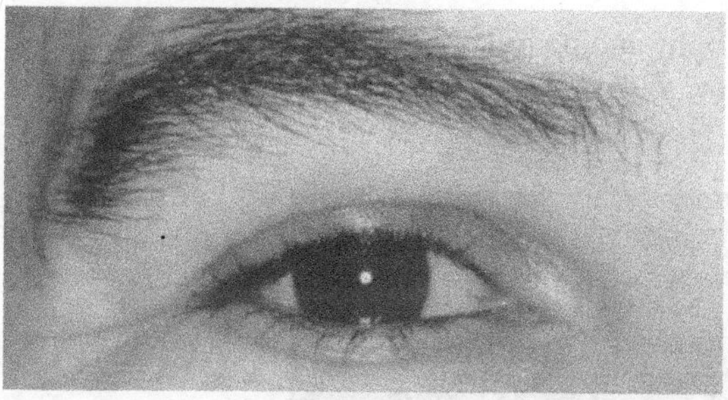

Figure 16 Blue sclera. Reproduced with permission of Aruna Dias from *Get Through MRCP Part 2: 350 Best of Fives*. London: RSM Press.

2. Age-related macular degeneration

On examination, there appear to be pale yellow spots in the macula, likely to be drusen. The diagnosis is age-related macular degeneration (ARMD). I would like to check the visual fields for a central scotoma.

What are drusen?

- They represent abnormal accumulations between the retinal pigment epithelium and basement (Bruch's) membrane (Figure 17):
  - drusen in the macular region lead to visual loss
  - there may be loss of central vision – examination may show a central scotoma

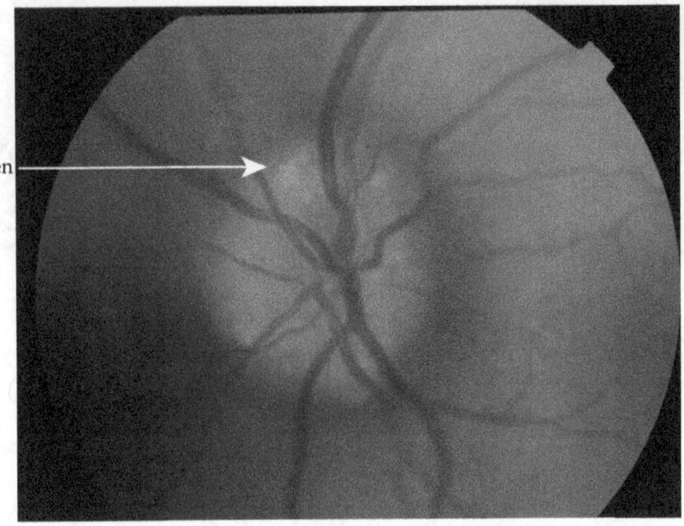

Figure 17 Drusen. Reproduced with permission of Eoin O'Sullivan.

What do you know about ARMD?

- There are two types:
  - dry type in which there is atrophy and no leakage of blood (Figure 18)
  - wet type in which there is neovascularization resulting in leakage of blood and visual loss (Figure 19)

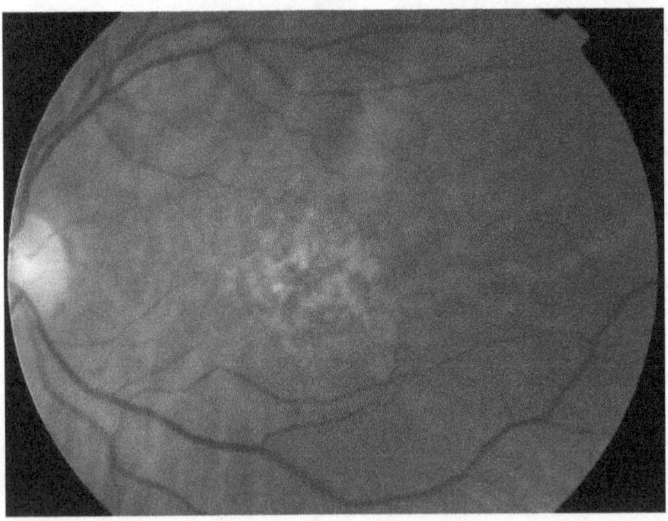

Figure 18 Dry macular degeneration. Reproduced with permission of Hiten G. Sheth.

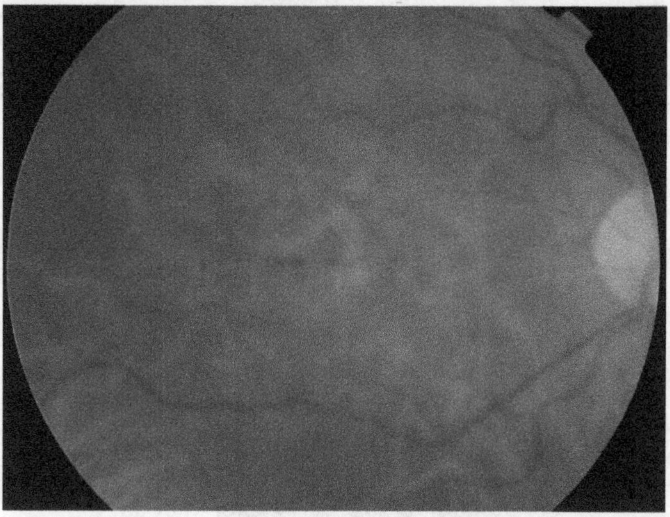

Figure 19 Wet macular degeneration. Reproduced with permission of Hiten G. Sheth.

How do you treat such patients?

Wet ARMD is treated with photocoagulation and surgery.

3. Papilloedema

On examination, there is swelling of the optic disc (Figure 20). I would like to check the visual fields to determine if there is enlargement of the blind spot. The diagnosis is papilloedema.

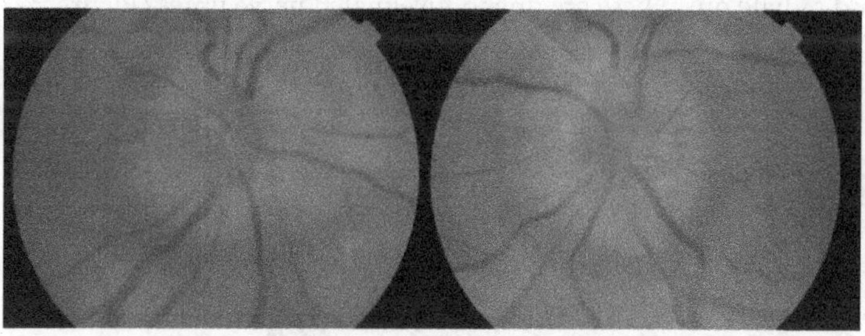

Figure 20 Papilloedema. Reproduced with permission of Eoin O'Sullivan.

NB Check carefully for hypertensive retinopathy.

What are the common causes of papilloedema?

- Hypertensive retinopathy
- Central retinal vein occlusion
- Benign intracranial hypertension
- Intracranial space-occupying lesion (look for associated CN VI palsy, which is a false localizing sign)

4. Glaucoma

On examination, the visual fields are constricted and the patient has only central vision. Fundoscopy shows cupping of the optic disc. The retina is not pigmented. The likely diagnosis is glaucoma (Figure 21).

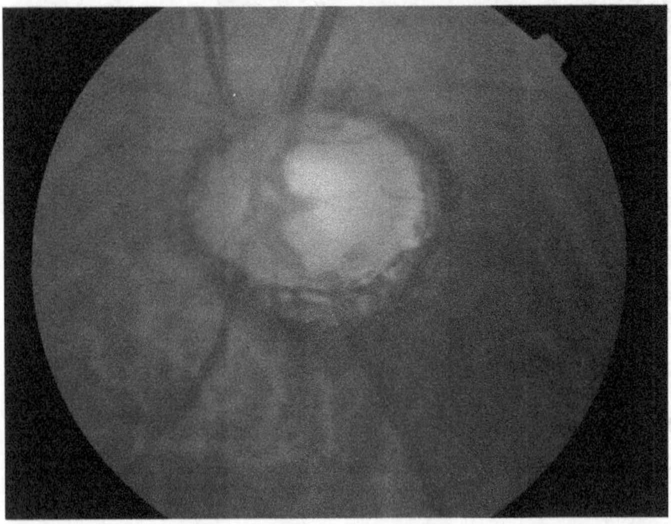

Figure 21 Glaucomatous disc. Reproduced with permission of Shamira Perera.

5. Myelinated nerve fibres

On examination, there are bright white, streaky, irregular patches which start at the edge of the disc and radiate out. These are due to myelinated nerve fibres (Figure 22) and do not affect vision.

Normally the fibres of the optic nerves lose their myelin sheath as they enter the eye. Occasionally the sheath persists for some distance after the fibres leave the optic disc.

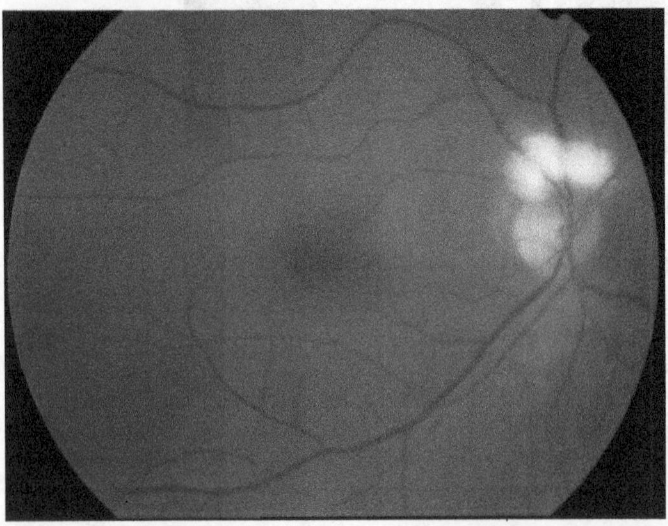

Figure 22 Myelinated nerve fibres. Reproduced with permission of Hiten G. Sheth.

6. Cataracts

On examination there is a cataract of the left (or right) eye (Figure 23).

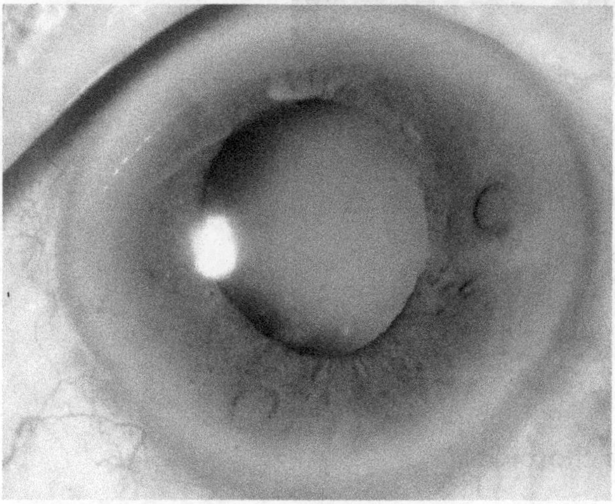

Figure 23 Cataract. Reproduced with permission of Shamira Perera.

What are the causes of cataracts?

- Old age
- Diabetes
- Myotonic dystrophy
- Hypoparathyroidism
- Radiation
- Steroids
- Hypoglycaemia
- Rubella

7. Old choroiditis

On examination there are patches of white and pigmented areas. White areas represent areas of atrophy and the pigmented areas represent areas of proliferation. The diagnosis is choroiditis (Figure 24).

NB Do not confuse with laser burns of diabetic retinopathy.

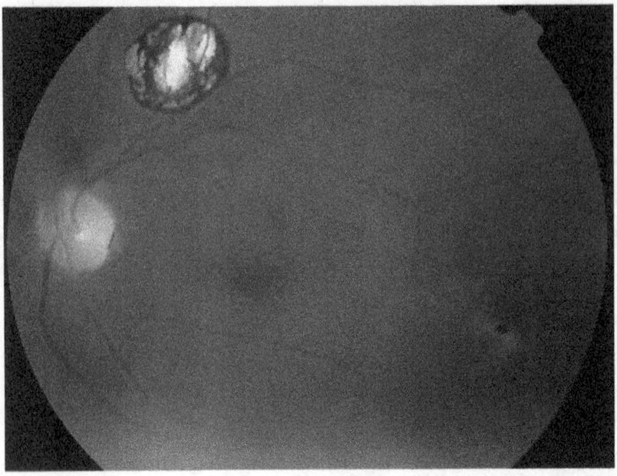

Figure 24 Old choroiditis. Reproduced with permission of Shamira Perera.

What are the causes of choroiditis?

- Toxoplasmosis
- Sarcoidosis
- AIDS
- Tuberculosis
- Syphilis
- Toxocariasis

8. Retinal artery occlusion

On examination, the retina is pale. There is a cherry red macula. The diagnosis is retinal artery occlusion (Figure 25). I would like to check the patient's vision as this condition is associated with sudden painless loss of vision.

NB The photograph shows a branch occlusion. The appearances are limited to one area and there is a corresponding field defect.

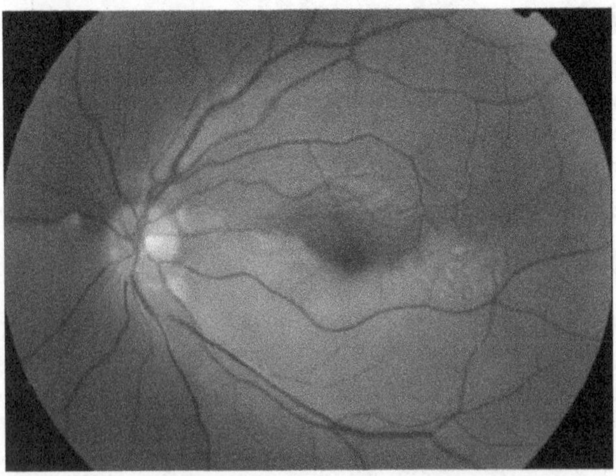

Figure 25 Branch retinal artery occlusion. Reproduced with permission from Hiten G. Sheth.

What are the common causes of retinal artery occlusion?

- AF
- Carotid stenosis
- Temporal arteritis
- Valvular heart disease

9. Retinal vein occlusion

On examination, the retinal veins are tortuous and dilated. There are flame haemorrhages, cotton wool spots and swelling of the optic disc (papilloedema). The diagnosis is central retinal vein occlusion.

NB: The findings may be restricted to one quadrant in branch retinal vein occlusion (Figure 26).

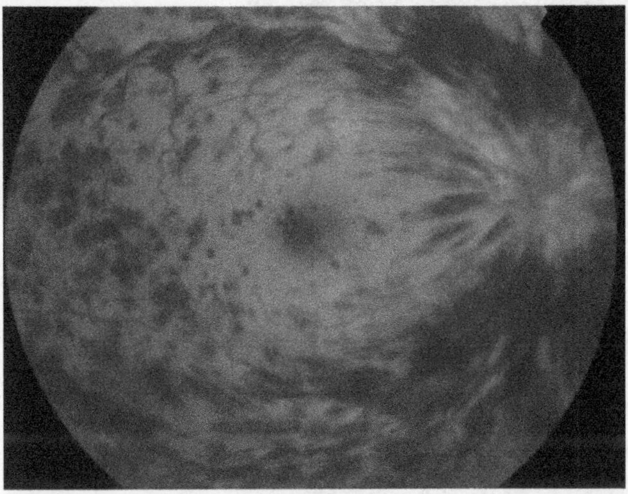

Figure 26 Central retinal vein occlusion. Reproduced with permission of Hiten G. Sheth.

What are the common causes of retinal vein occlusion?

- Diabetes
- Hypertension
- Glaucoma
- Hyperviscosity with Waldenström's macroglobulinaemia, myeloma, or PRV
- Vasculitis

What treatment options are available?

- Treat the underlying condition
- Pan-retinal photocoagulation to prevent the neovascular complications of rubeosis iridis and rubeosis glaucoma

DERMATOLOGY

10. Kaposi's sarcoma

Describe the skin lesion

These are violaceous/purple raised plaques/nodules on the skin, which may occur alone or in crops and can occur on the limbs, mucous membranes or anywhere else on the skin.

This is consistent with Kaposi's sarcoma (Figure 27).

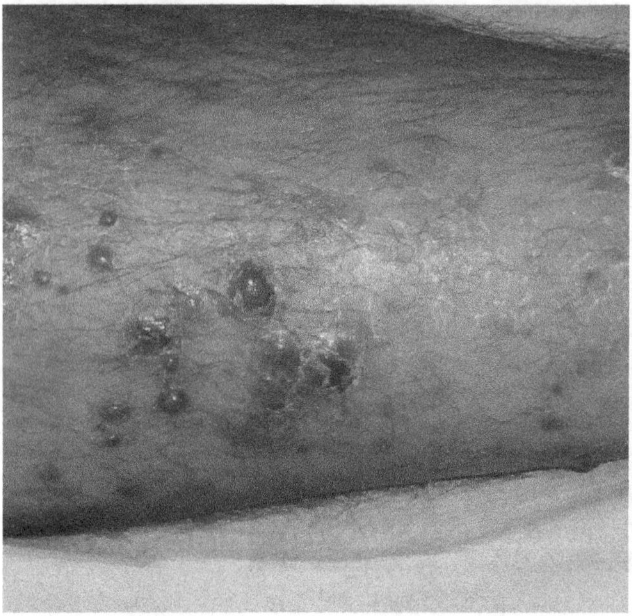

Figure 27 Kaposi's sarcoma. Reproduced with permission of Begoña Bovill.

What questions might you ask this patient?

Find out if he or she has any immunodeficiencies, e.g. HIV positive, or is on immunosuppressive drug therapy following an organ transplant.

What is the aetiology?

In this patient it is human herpesvirus 8 (an AIDS-defining illness).

Describe the different types of Kaposi's sarcoma

AIDS defining

- Poor prognosis
- Commonly associated with haematological malignancies and secondary infection

African Kaposi's

- Aggressive sarcoma
- Poor prognosis

Classic variety

- Occurring in Jewish men and those of Mediterranean origin
- Peripheral distribution
- Good prognosis

Immunodeficiency related

- Particularly on therapy after organ transplantation
- Majority are Afro-Caribbean
- May resolve when immunosuppression reduced

Discuss the complications of Kaposi's sarcoma

- Visceral involvement – commonly gastrointestinal involvement
- Metastases to lymph nodes
- Lymphatic obstruction and cellulitis

What investigations would you conduct in this patient?

- Bloods – FBC, blood film looking for associated haematological malignancies
- HIV testing
- Skin biopsy (histology: spindle-shaped cells, slit-like spaces filled with red cells)

What is the management of this condition?

- Treat underlying cause, e.g. antiretroviral drugs
- If systemic, consider radiotherapy, interferon, chemotherapy
- Consider underlying causes, e.g. reduction of immunosuppressive treatment

11. Basal cell carcinoma

Describe this lesion

It is located on the face (usually on sun exposed areas of the body). Its surface has telangiectasia, there is central ulceration and rolled raised margins (often start off as a 'pearly papule').

This is consistent with a BCC (Figure 28).

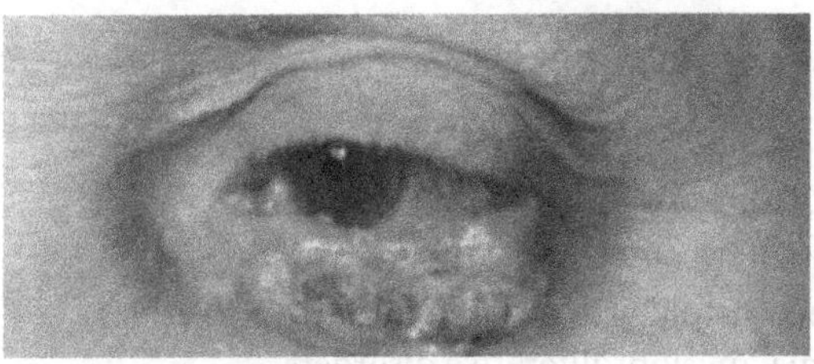

Figure 28 BCC. Reproduced with permission of Aruna Dias from *Get Through MRCP Part 2: 350 Best of Fives*. London: RSM Press.

Describe the growth and spread of a BCC

- They often follow a slow growth pattern and rarely spread or metastasize.

What groups of patients are more likely to have this condition?

- It is commonest in the elderly and fair-skinned individuals.

What types of BCC do you know?

- Superficial
- Nodular
- Morphoeic
- Pigmented

How would you treat this condition?

Treatment options include:

- Excision (Mohs surgery for critical sites)
- Cryotherapy
- Radiotherapy
- Curettage

12. Pyoderma gangrenosum

Describe this lesion

There is a necrotic ulcer with a ragged purple coloured overhanging edge. This is located on the leg (although it can occur anywhere on the body).

The patient has pyoderma gangrenosum (Figure 29).

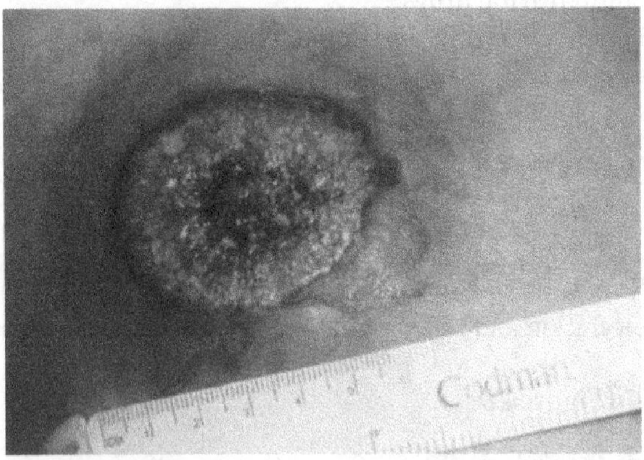

Figure 29 Pyoderma gangrenosum. Reproduced with permission of Aruna Dias from *Get Through MRCP Part 2: 350 Best of Fives*. London: RSM Press.

Name some causes of this condition

- Inflammatory bowel disease (50% have ulcerative colitis)
- Autoimmune conditions (e.g. rheumatoid arthritis, seronegative arthritides)
- Lymphomas/leukaemias, myeloma, myeloproliferative disorders
- Chronic active hepatitis

Describe the pathogenesis

Pyoderma gangrenosum is thought to arise as a result of immune system dysfunction, in particular a problem with neutrophils. The condition is, however, poorly understood.

How would you treat this condition?

- Treat the underlying cause
- Local treatments – intralesional steroids, dressings
- Systemic treatments – oral steroids, dapsone, tetracyclines

13. Malignant melanoma

Describe the lesions

For example, there is a solitary lesion on the cheek, 25 mm wide, which has varying pigmentation with different colours and an irregular border. There is some inflammation on the surrounding skin but no satellite lesions. I would like to check the local lymph nodes and the liver.

These findings are consistent with melanoma (Figure 30).

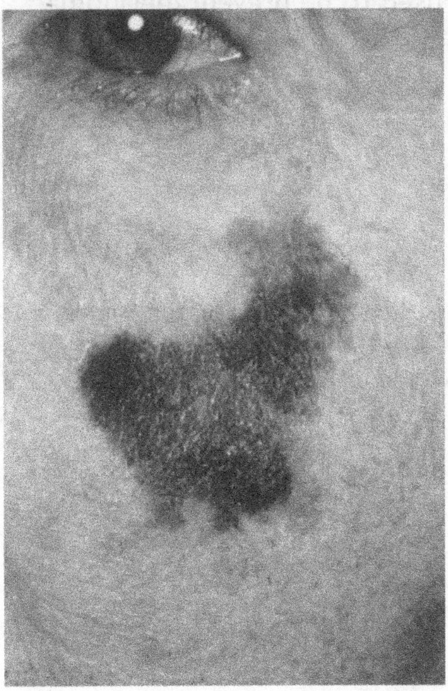

Figure 30 Malignant melanoma. Reproduced with permission of Aruna Dias from *Get Through MRCP Part 2: 350 Best of Fives*. London: RSM Press.

Discuss the various types of melanoma

- Lentigo maligna: located on sun-exposed areas, commonest in the elderly, risk of malignant transformation

- Superficial spreading: most common type. Tends to grow horizontally across epidermal and superficial epidermal planes (radial growth) and not reach lymphatics and blood vessels so prognosis tends to be good
- Acral lentiginous: confined to palms, soles and nails
- Nodular: growth is in the vertical plane, tends to be dome shaped, poor prognosis
- Amelanotic

What are the main determinants of poor prognosis in melanoma?

- Depth of invasion is the most important factor. The thickness of the tumour beneath the epidermis (Breslow's thickness) correlates inversely with prognosis
- Spread to regional lymph nodes
- Presence of metastases
- Ulceration

How would you treat this condition?

- Excision of 2 mm healthy skin margin. After histology, wider excision is carried out
- Sentinel node biopsy – to determine local spread which helps determine treatment and prognosis

What preventative methods can be used to be prevent melanoma?

Reducing exposure to the sun, using high-factor sunscreen and wearing protective clothing.

14. Bullous pemphigoid

Describe the lesions

There are tense, clear (can be blood-stained) blisters on the arms. They vary in size up to few centimetres in diameter. I would like to examine the mucous membranes (usually spared in pemphigoid).

This is consistent with bullous pemphigoid (Figure 31).

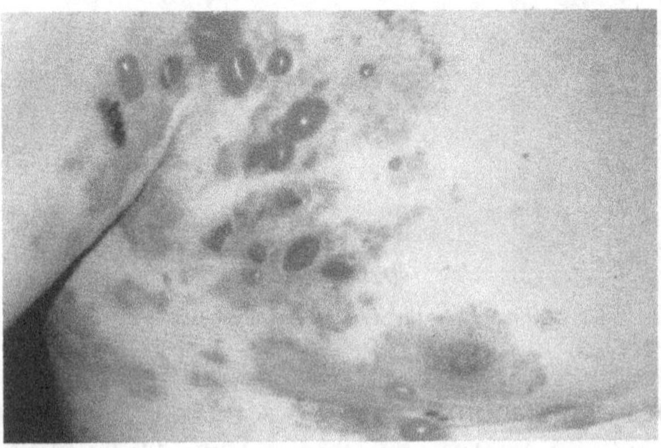

Figure 31 Bullous pemphigoid. Reproduced with permission of Aruna Dias from *Get Through MRCP Part 2: 350 Best of Fives*. London: RSM Press.

What particular features would you like to elicit in the history?

- Age (usually affects the elderly)
- Natural history of condition – can start with vague localized rash, which after several weeks becomes more generalized. It tends to involve the limbs and trunk
- Drug history
- Involvement of mucosal surfaces

Discuss the pathogenesis of this condition

- This is a subepidermal blistering autoimmune condition.
- IgG and C3 complement are found in the basement membrane.

How would you confirm this condition?

- Skin biopsy

What is the other main bullous disease?

Pemphigus vulgaris is another blistering condition characterized by autoimmune destruction of the epidermal layer (Figure 32). IgG antibodies target keratinocytes. It is commonest in Jews and tends to affect the middle aged and elderly. There are initially eroded lesions appearing in the mucous membranes; this then progresses to involve the skin. One of the key clinical features is Nikolsky's sign (separation of the epidermal layer after applying pressure laterally over the blister).

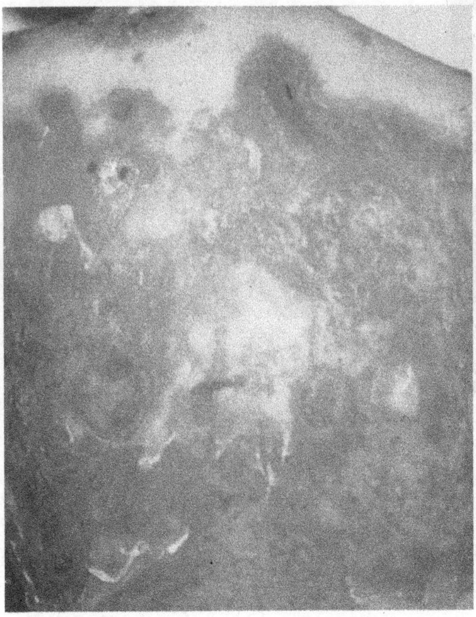

Figure 32 Pemphigus vulgaris. Reproduced with permission of Aruna Dias from *Get Through MRCP Part 2: 350 Best of Fives*. London: RSM Press.

How would you manage this patient?

- Steroids and immunosuppressive treatments, e.g. azathioprine
- The condition often occurs in relapses and remissions

List other bullous diseases

- Dermatitis herpetiformis
- Epidermolysis bullosa
- Linear IgA disease
- Herpes gestationis

15. Erythema multiforme

Describe the lesions

There are many blisters, which are inside at least one ring, so-called target lesions. These are on the palms of the hand, but can also occur on the arms, dorsum of the feet and the knees. I would also like to examine the mucous membranes (for Stevens–Johnson syndrome) and genitalia (there may also be bullae and papules)

This is consistent with erythema multiforme (Figure 33).

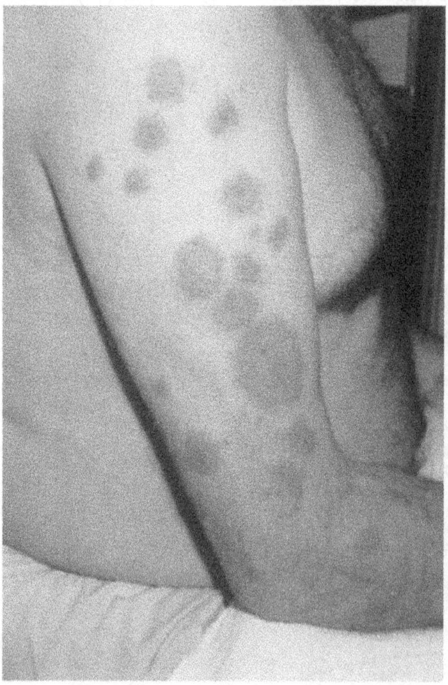

Figure 33 Erythema multiforme. Reproduced with permission of Aruna Dias from *Get Through MRCP Part 2: 350 Best of Fives*. London: RSM Press.

What are the causes of this condition?

- Idiopathic – 50%
- Infection – viral (e.g. herpes simplex), bacterial (streptococcal throat, mycoplasma)
- Drugs – penicillin, NSAIDs, sulfonamides
- Vaccinations
- Connective tissue diseases, e.g. SLE
- Neoplastic – carcinoma, lymphoma, myeloma

What are the complications?

- Stevens–Johnson syndrome – potentially fatal
- Eye – corneal ulcers, conjunctivitis, uveitis
- Toxic epidermolysis necrosis (TEN)

How would you manage this condition?

- It is usually self-limiting

Supportive

- Oral toilet
- Rehydration
- Analgesia
- Ophthalmology input if there are eye complications

Medical

- Treat underlying cause
- Antibiotics/aciclovir
- Consider steroids
- Immunosuppression used rarely
- Stop offending drugs
- Burns unit or ICU for severe cases or TEN

16. Purpura

Describe these skin lesions

There are well-defined, bright red lesions distributed symmetrically on the legs. They do not blanch with pressure. I would like to examine this patient for signs of lymphadenopathy, hepatomegaly and splenomegaly, as well as inspect for any underlying causes.

The patient has purpuric lesions (Figure 34).

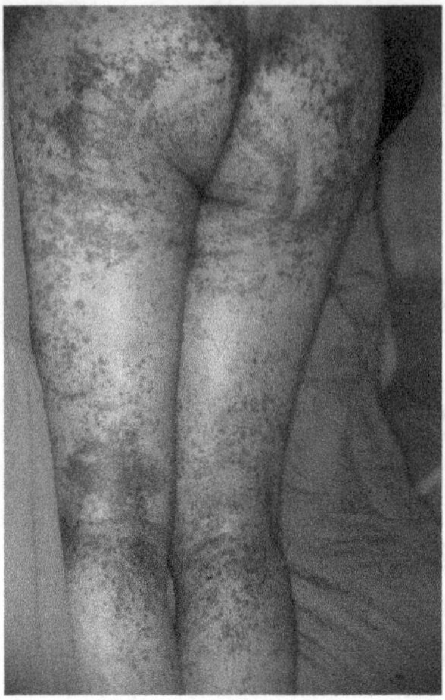

Figure 34 Purpura. Reproduced with permission of Begoña Bovill.

What is the pathogenesis of such lesions?

They are due to red cells leaking into the surrounding skin from blood vessels. Causes can be thrombocytopaenic, vascular or due to clotting defects.

What are the causes?

Thrombocytopaenic

- Idiopathic thrombocytopaenic purpura
- Haematological disorders: leukaemias, any cause of bone marrow failure
- Drugs: rifampicin, cytotoxics, gold
- Septicaemia

Vascular

- Senile purpura
- Henoch–Schönlein purpura
- Drugs: steroids, carbimazole, thiazides
- Cutaneous vasculitis (due to infection, autoimmune conditions, drugs)
- Scurvy

Clotting defects

- Drugs: e.g. warfarin
- Haemophilia
- Christmas disease
- von Willebrand's disease

Tell me about Henoch–Schönlein purpura

- Commonest in children
- Type of vasculitis, characterized by purpuric lesions over the buttocks and extensor aspects of the lower limbs
- Also can be associated with arthritis, gastrointestinal bleeding and nephritis

17. Acanthosis nigricans

Describe the lesion

This is a soft, velvety, brown/hyperpigmented lesion located in the axillary region (can also present on other body-fold areas).

The patient has acanthosis nigricans (Figure 35).

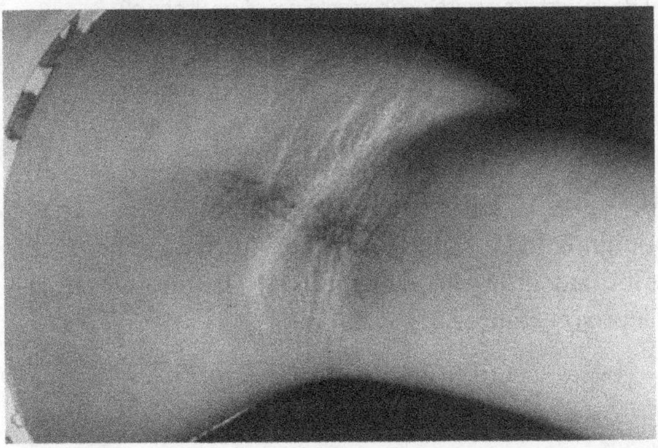

Figure 35 Acanthosis nigricans. Reproduced with permission of Aruna Dias from *Get Through MRCP Part 2: 350 Best of Fives*. London: RSM Press.

What is the most serious underlying condition you would like to rule out?

An adenocarcinoma (most often affecting the stomach, intestinal tract or uterus).

Which other conditions is this skin lesion associated with?

Endocrine disorders

- Diabetes
- Obesity
- Cushing's
- Acromegaly
- Polycystic ovaries
- Hyper- and hypothyroidism

Malignancy

- Ovarian
- Breast

- Prostate
- Rarely lymphomas

Discuss some other cutaneous manifestations of malignancy

Table 18 Cutaneous manifestations of malignancy

Dermatomyositis	bronchial and breast carcinoma
Paget's disease of the nipple	intraductal carcinoma
Clubbing	bronchial carcinoma
Icthyosis	lymphomas
Necrotic migratory erythema	pancreatic tumours (especially glucagon-secreting tumours)
Bowen's disease	SCC of the skin
Genetic disorders	neurofibromatosis, Wiscott–Aldrich syndrome (lymphomas), Peutz–Jeghers syndrome (hamartomas of small bowel)

18. Leprosy

Describe the salient clinical findings in this patient

This patient has flattened hypopigmented macules located on the back. There is also a thickened ulnar nerve located at the medial left elbow. The findings are consistent with a diagnosis of leprosy (Figure 36).

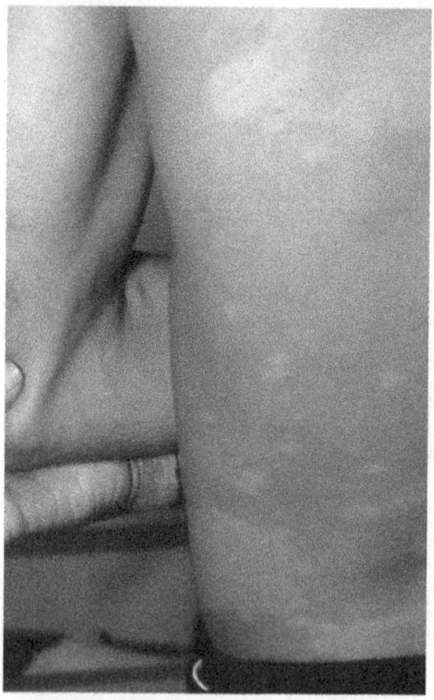

Figure 36 Leprosy. Reproduced with permission of Begoña Bovill.

What investigations would you want to do to confirm your diagnosis?

- Skin-slit smears or biopsy looking for acid-fast bacilli. This case is more typical of a tuberculoid leprosy rather than a lepromatous leprosy, in which nerve damage is rare.

What is the treatment for leprosy?

- Patient education, e.g. prevention of skin ulcers
- Physiotherapy for ulcers and deformities
- According to WHO guidelines, the treatment regime for tuberculoid leprosy and borderline leprosy lasts for 6 months and consists of:
  - rifampicin 600 mg once a month *and*
  - dapsone 100 mg o.d.
- For lepromatous leprosy, borderline leprosy and borderline lepromatous leprosy, the treatment regime lasts for 12 months and consists of:
  - rifampicin 600 mg once a month
  - clofazimine 300 mg once a month
  - dapsone 100 mg o.d.

19. Splinter haemorrhages

Describe the abnormalities

There are small, subungual linear haemorrhages (Figure 37).

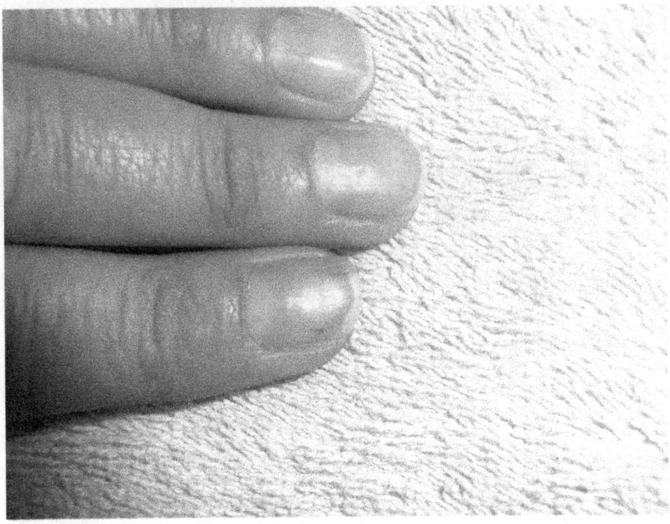

Figure 37 Splinter haemorrhages. Reproduced with permission of Begoña Bovill.

What are the causes of splinter haemorrhages?

- Trauma – commonest cause
- Infective endocarditis

20. Clubbing

Describe this abnormality

There is increased longitudinal and transverse curvature of the nail, the nail bed has a spongy consistency and the nail bed is swollen. These changes are consistent with clubbing (Figure 38).

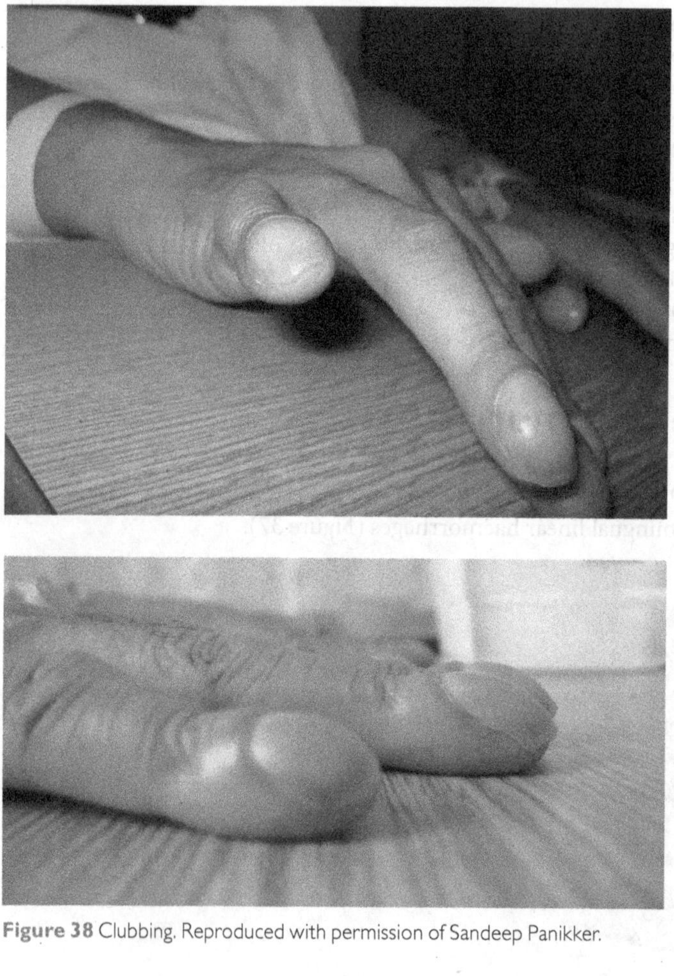

Figure 38 Clubbing. Reproduced with permission of Sandeep Panikker.

What are the causes of clubbing?

Respiratory

- Bronchial carcinoma
- Fibrosing alveolitis
- Bronchiectasis
- Lung empyema

Cardiac

- Congenital cyanotic heart disease
- Infective endocarditis

Gastrointestinal

- Inflammatory bowel disease
- Cirrhotic liver disease

II

CHAPTER 2 EXAMINATION SKILLS

Examination of the skin

- The skin station may consist of an individual skin lesion or a rash (multiple lesions). The approach to these is different, so we have categorized this section into these two types. For the purposes of the exam you should still follow basic principles. One approach is to LOOK, FEEL AND MOVE.
- It is important to describe the skin lesion with the appropriate terminology and then give your differential diagnoses.
- Begin with a general evaluation of the exposed patient.

Description of an individual lump or a single skin lesion

- Anatomical site
- Number of lesions, e.g. satellite lesions in malignant melanoma and Merkel cell carcinoma
- Surface – macule/papule/nodule, ulcerated, hyperkeratotic, smooth, scaly, blisters
- Colour and pigmentation – several colours may be present in malignant melanoma
- Border – is it well demarcated or are the margins irregular or diffuse?
- Size – measure if a ruler is available
- Consistency – ask about tenderness first!
    - soft and fluctuant in lipoma, cyst or abscess
    - attachment to surrounding tissue
- Surrounding tissue – erythema, induration, sun damage, excoriation marks
- Other features – pulsatile or presence of bruit
- Check other body sites, if relevant, such as lymph nodes, mucosal surfaces and nails (for example in psoriasis)

Description of rashes (multiple skin lesions)

- Distribution – bilateral, symmetrical, flexural, extensor surfaces, sun-exposed areas, presence in surgical scars
- Appearance of individual lesions (as above)
- Check nails, scalp and mucous membranes
- Remember many skin conditions are manifestations of systemic disease such as autoimmune disease, so look for general clues – exophthalmos for thyroid disease and cushingoid features

Examination of the cardiovascular system

Initial steps

- Introduce yourself and ask for consent to examine the patient.
- Expose the patient's precordium.
- Sit the patient at 45 degrees and make sure that he or she is comfortable.

Inspection

General inspection

- Check around the bedside for cigarettes, oxygen cylinder or GTN spray.
- Note if the patient is short of breath.
- Note any scars such as a midline sternotomy or left axillary scar.
- Check for signs of systemic diseases such as Cushing's or Marfan's disease.

Hands

- Clubbing, which is found in congenital cyanotic heart disease, infective endocarditis and atrial myxoma
- Splinter haemorrhages, which result from infective endocarditis or trauma
- Check capillary refill time to check perfusion
- Check for peripheral cyanosis
- Check for nicotine staining of fingers
- Osler's nodes – found in infective endocarditis
- Janeway lesions – found in infective endocarditis
- Tendon xanthomata – found in familial hypercholesterolaemia

Pulse

- Rate – bradycardia suggests β-blocker use or a conduction defect while tachycardia may be present in AF
- Rhythm – irregular in AF
- Volume – high volume pulse in hyperdynamic circulation from pregnancy, anaemia, thyrotoxicosis, aortic regurgitation. Small volume in aortic stenosis (best checked for at the carotid artery)
- Collapsing pulse – in aortic regurgitation
- Check for radiofemoral and radioradial delay, which are present in coarctation of the aorta
- Check the brachial and carotid pulses and offer to check all other peripheral pulses

Face

- Malar flush of mitral stenosis
- Eyes for xanthelasma or corneal arcus
- Mouth for central cyanosis, high arched palate (Marfan's disease)

Neck

- Inspect the JVP
- Inspect for any visible carotid pulsations – in aortic regurgitation

Palpation

Apex beat

- Check for displacement from the fifth intercostal space, mid-clavicular line
- Feel for character, e.g. tapping apex (mitral stenosis), jerky pulse (HOCM), collapsing pulse (aortic regurgitation, PDA, AV fistula)

Precordium

- Parasternal heaves (in hypertrophy of ventricle and atria)
- Thrills (palpable murmur)

Auscultation

- Listen to the heart sounds:
  - palpate the carotid pulse simultaneously in order to time the heart sounds
  - work systematically in the following order: mitral, tricuspid, pulmonary and aortic
  - listen for the first and second heart sounds, loudness of heart sounds (soft first heart sound in mitral regurgitation and soft second heart sound in aortic stenosis), third and fourth heart sounds
- Listen for murmurs:
  - comment on the timing and type of murmur (ejection systolic, pansystolic, early diastolic, etc.)
  - accentuate the murmur – left-sided murmurs are best heard in held expiration; right-sided murmurs are best heard in held inspiration; mitral murmurs are best heard in the left lateral position; aortic murmurs are best heard with the patient leaning forwards
  - radiation to carotid arteries or back
- Auscultate the carotids for bruits.
- Listen to the lung bases for crepitations of pulmonary oedema.
- Percuss the lung bases if suspecting effusion.

Ankles

- Check for sacral oedema and ankle swelling.

On completion

- Offer to:
  - check the blood pressure
  - dipstick the urine for microscopic haematuria (infective endocarditis)
  - check the temperature chart
  - palpate the abdomen for hepatomegaly, splenomegaly and ascites

Examination of the nervous system

Cranial nerves

CN I

- Enquire about any change in smell.
- Offer to test each nostril with essence bottles.

CN II

- Test acuity with corrected lenses using a Snellen chart.
- Examine the direct and consensual reflex (consensual reflex is testing CN III).
- Check accommodation.
- Test visual fields.
- Test colour vision.
- Perform fundoscopy for optic atrophy, papilloedema and retinal examination.

CNs III, IV and VI

- Inspect pupils for size.
- Inspect for signs of palsy:
  - CN III: characteristic down and out eyeball, dilated pupil, ptosis
  - CN IV: unable to look down and in, may hold head on a tilt
  - CN VI: eye is turned inwards, unable to move outwards.
- Look for ptosis.
- Check ocular movements to look for nystagmus and diplopia.

CN V

- Test sensation (light touch and pin prick) in ophthalmic, maxillary and mandibular divisions.
- Offer to test temperature sensation.
- Ask patient to open mouth and clench teeth to test masseter muscles.
- Test jaw jerk reflex.
- Palpate masseter and temporal muscles for signs of wasting.
- Offer to test corneal reflex.

CN VII

- Inspect for facial asymmetry – look for loss of nasolabial folds and forehead creases.
- Examine power of facial muscles (complete ipsilateral weakness suggests LMN lesion while sparing of frontalis muscle indicates UMN lesion):
  - test eyelid strength
  - ask patient to raise eyebrows
  - ask patient to grin and blow out checks
  - ask the patient to show his/her teeth

CN VIII

- Establish that there is a hearing problem.
- Whisper a word into each ear and ask the patient to repeat back.
- Ask the patient if he or she can hear the ticking hands of a watch.
- If there is a hearing impairment picked up, then carry out Weber's and Rinne's tests to establish if is conductive or sensorineural.

Weber's test – tests bone conduction only

- Test by placing the activated tuning fork on the middle of the forehead and then asking the patient in which ear the sound is heard loudest. If heard in both ears equally loudly, the test is normal.
- If there is conductive hearing loss, then the sound is heard loudest in the defective ear.
- If there is sensorineual hearing loss, then the sound is heard loudest in the 'good' ear.

Rinne's test – tests air conduction (AC) and bone conduction (BC)

- Place the tuning fork on the mastoid process of one ear (testing BC) until the sound is no longer heard. At this point place the tuning fork in front of the ear (testing AC).
- If AC > BC, this could be normal or there could be sensorineural deafness in that ear. Weber's test will help you make this distinction.
- If there is conductive hearing loss, then BC > AC.

CNs IX and X

- Examine the palate for uvular deviation; the uvula is drawn to normal side if the lesion is unilateral.
- Ask patient to say 'Ah' to test palatal movement.
- Offer to check gag reflex (CNs IX and X).

CN XI

- Examine strength of trapezius and sternocleidomastoid muscles.

CN XII

- Examine tongue for wasting and fasciculation.
- Ask patient to stick the tongue out – the tongue projects towards the affected side if there is a lesion.
- Test tongue strength against cheek.

Eyes

- The list below outlines the systematic way of approaching examination of the eyes.
- You may be asked to perform one component of this examination, e.g. 'examine the visual fields in this patient'.
- Be guided by your initial inspection of the patient.

General inspection

- Stand back and have a look at the patient to try to generally assess whether he or she has any signs of systemic disease that might be associated with eye problems, such as acromegaly, hyperthyroidism or diabetes.
- Have a close look at the whole face:
  - facial asymmetry (due to CN VIII UMN lesion associated with homonymous hemianopia)
  - acromegaly (associated with bitemporal hemianopia)

External eyes

- Examine the eyelids:
  - xanthalesma
  - ptosis, which may be caused by CN III palsy, Horner's syndrome, myasthenia gravis or myotonic dystrophy
- Examine the position of the eyeball, looking for:
  - strabismus
  - down and out eyeball in CN III palsy
  - any signs of CN IV or CN VI palsy
  - proptosis – exophthlamos in thyroid eye disease
- Inspect the sclera and conjunctiva for corneal arcus and Keyser–Fleischer rings.

Pupils

- Size:
  - small pupil, e.g. Argyll Robertson pupil, Horner's syndrome
  - large pupil, e.g. CN III palsy, Holmes–Adie syndrome
- Pupillary reflexes
  - direct and consensual reflexes using the swinging flashlight test
  - accommodation

Assess visual acuity

- Use a Snellen chart.

Visual fields

- Hemianopia
  - homonymous hemianopia following a stroke
  - bitemporal hemianopia – lesion at optic chiasm, e.g. pituitary tumour
- Quadrantanopia
- Central scotoma

Eye movements

- Examine cranial nerve palsies:
  - down and out pupil – CN III palsy
  - weakness in downward movement – CN IV palsy
  - unable to move eye laterally – CN VI palsy

- Look for horizontal and vertical nystagmus:
  - presents in cerebellar disease
- Enquire about diplopia:
  - occurs at the extremes of the gaze
  - ask the patient to state the presence of an outer and inner image
  - ask the patient to cover one eye – when the outer image disappears the covered eye is the one with the pathology

Fundoscopy

- Check presence of red reflex – may be absent with cataract.
- Assess the optic disc:
  - optic atrophy
  - papilloedema
- Assess the macula:
  - cherry red spot
  - pallor
  - exudates
- Retinal inspection:
  - diabetic retinopathy
  - hypertensive retinopathy
  - retinitis pigmentosa

Cerebellar system

General inspection

- Have a general look at the patient. Look for walking aids
- UMN lesion and cerebellar signs indicate a brainstem lesion

Remember: DANISH

- **D**ysdiadochokinesis
- **A**taxia:
  - falling towards side of lesion
  - truncal ataxia (vermis lesion)
  - heel–shin ataxia
- **N**ystagmus
- **I**ntention tremor, past-pointing and resting tremor
- **S**taccato speech
- **H**ypotonia/hyper-reflexia

Tests of coordination

Upper limbs

- Intention tremor and past pointing:
  - ask the patient to touch your finger with their index finger and then touch their nose
  - place your hand at arms length and ask the patient to repeat a few times, asking them to carry out the action faster

- repeat for opposite side
- watch out for intention tremor and past pointing
- Dysdiadochokinesis – ask the patient to tap the palm of the left hand alternately with the palm and dorsum of the right hand. Ask them to repeat and carry this out faster as they get used to it. Repeat for the other side.

Lower limbs

- Heel–shin ataxia:
  - With the patient lying down, ask the patient to place their right ankle on their left knee and slide down the leg to the ankle, move the right foot in the air, back on to the left knee and repeat – ask them to do this a few times, speeding up if they can
  - repeat for the opposite side
  - watch out for heel–shin ataxia
- Test for truncal ataxia by asking the patient sit down with the arms folded. If there is truncal ataxia the patient will sway from side to side. The truncal ataxic gait is described fully on p. 122.

Romberg's test

- This tests for proprioception and sensory ataxia.
- The test is carried out in two stages:
  - Ask the patient to stand up straight, with the feet together. Patients with cerebellar disease will not be able to stay balanced at this stage
  - Ask the patient to close their eyes. If the patient begins to sway or topple once the eyes are closed, then the test is positive
- Stand next to the patient, ready to act in case they fall.
- A positive test indicates a sensory ataxia. It is not a test of cerebellar function.
- Conditions causing a positive result are diseases of the dorsal columns and peripheral neuropathies.

Peripheral nervous system – upper and lower limbs

General inspection

- Look for cachexia, signs of facial weakness, tremor or obvious neurological deficit.
- Look for muscle wasting in the various muscle groups.
- Look for distribution of weakness, e.g. pyramidal weakness in patients who have had a CVA.
- Inspect for fasciculation.
- Look for scarring.
- Look for any deformities.

Tone

- Ask the patient to go floppy in the limbs and move the limbs at the knees/elbows with rolling as well as flexion/extension movements.
- The patient should be lying down for lower limb examination but can be lying or sitting for upper limb examination.
- Check for clonus in the ankles and wrists.
- Tone is increased in UMN lesions.

- Tone is reduced or flaccid in LMN lesions or cerebellar lesions.
- Also look out for characteristic tone, e.g. cogwheel and lead pipe rigidity, spastic tone (clasp knife).

Power

- Test all muscle groups in the upper and lower limbs.
- Start proximally and move distally.
- In the lower limbs check for:
  - hip flexion (ileopsoas), extension and abduction (glutei), adduction (adductors)
  - knee flexion (hamstrings) and extension (quadriceps)
  - ankle dorsiflexion (tibialis anterior and long extensors), plantar flexion (gastrocnemius), eversion (peronei) and inversion (tibialis anterior and posterior)
- In the upper limbs check for:
  - shoulder abduction (deltoids), adduction (pectoralis)
  - elbow flexion (biceps), extension (triceps)
  - wrist flexion and extension
- Grading:
  - 5 = normal power
  - 4 = reduced power but can still maintain position against resistance
  - 3 = movement against gravity but not resistance
  - 2 = movement but not against gravity
  - 1 = flicker/mild contraction
  - 0 = no movement

Reflexes

Upper limbs
- Supinator (C5/6)
- Biceps (C5/6)
- Triceps (C7/8)

Lower limbs
- Ankle (S1/2)
- Knee (L3/4)
- Feet for plantar (Babinski's) reflex – if positive, suggests upper motor neuron lesion

Sensation

- Check each dermatome.
- Check for sensory level especially in the lower limbs.

What to examine for
- Light touch sensation – carried in dorsal columns and spinothalamic tracts
- Dorsal columns:
  - joint position sense – in the great toes

- vibration sense – compare with vibration sense on sternum first: for lower limbs start distally at metatarsal head and move proximally to malleolus, knee, iliac crest; for upper limb check distal IPJ, proximal IPJ, wrist, elbow, shoulder
- Spinothalamic tract:
  - pain – examine pin-prick sensation by examining the difference between the sharp and blunt ends; test in a dermatomal distribution starting distally and moving proximally
  - temperature sensation – offer to check hot and cold sensation; test as for pain sensation

On completion

Tell the examiner you would like to finish your examination by assessing the function of the cranial nerves, checking for cerebellar lesions and completing the peripheral nerve examination.

Examination of the abdominal system

Initial steps

- Introduce yourself to the patient and ask for consent to examine them.
- Expose the patient from the xiphisternum to the pubic symphysis.
- Position the patient so they are lying flat on the bed comfortably with a single pillow to support their head and with their arms by their sides.

Inspection

Skin

- Skin colour:
  - jaundice suggesting liver failure
  - pallor suggesting anaemia
  - hyperpigmentation with haemochromatosis or uraemia
- Scratch marks suggesting pruritus

Hands

- Clubbing is found in IBD, coeliac disease and liver cirrhosis.
- Leuconychia due to hypoalbuminaemia is found in chronic liver disease or renal failure.
- Koilonychia is due to iron deficiency, which can occur with chronic blood loss.
- Palmar erythema is seen in chronic liver disease.
- Dupuytren's contracture is seen with liver cirrhosis.
- Asterixis or a hepatic flap suggests liver failure.

Arms

- Arteriovenous fistula suggests renal failure.
- Tattoos suggest the possibility of hepatitis C.
- Needle marks from intravenous drug use suggest the possibility of hepatitis C.

Face

- Kayser–Fleischer rings are seen in Wilson's disease.
- Sclera can show anaemia or jaundice.
- Xanthelasma around the eyelids is seen in PBC.
- Mouth ulcers are found in Crohn's disease.
- Peri-oral hyperpigmentation is seen in Peutz–Jeghers disease.

Neck

- Supraclavicular and cervical lymph nodes

Chest

- Spider naevi
- Gynaecomastia

Abdomen

- Localized or generalized swellings, scars from gastrointestinal surgery or renal transplant
- Abnormal pulsations from an abdominal aortic aneurysm
- Caput medusa – veins radiating from the umbilicus due to portal hypertension

Palpation

- Check whether the patient has any abdominal pain or discomfort.
- Kneel at the bedside and palpate the abdomen at the same level with the pulp of your fingers.
- While palpating look at the patient's face to see if he or she grimaces, suggesting that the area is tender.
- Palpate all nine regions:
  - left hypochondrium, left flank, left iliac fossa
  - epigastrium, umbilical area, hypogastrium
  - right hypochondrium, right flank and right iliac fossa
- Start superficially, then palpate deeply.

Mass

- Determine:
  - location
  - size
  - shape
  - surface
  - whether it is pulsatile
  - whether it moves with respiration

Liver

- The liver enlarges from below the right costal margin downwards. Therefore, start to palpate for the liver from the right iliac fossa.

- Hepatomegaly should be measured in centimetres from below the costal margin.
- Describe the liver edge:
  - smooth edge: healthy individuals, hepatitis, heart failure
  - nodular edge: malignancy (usually metastases; rarely primary), cirrhosis of the liver
  - pulsatile liver: tricuspid regurgitation
  - tender edge: hepatitis, cardiac failure

Spleen

- The spleen enlarges from below the left costal margin towards the right iliac fossa.
- Therefore, start to palpate for the spleen from the right iliac fossa.
- Ask the patient to roll on to his or her right side to detect splenomegaly.

Kidneys

- Use bimanual palpation and ballottement.
- Be gentle if there is a mass in the iliac fossa as this may be a transplanted kidney.
- Note whether the kidney is ballottable, you can get over it and there is no notch.

Other areas

- Check groin for lymph nodes.
- Check for hernia orifices.
- Check for the expansile pulsation of an aortic aneurysm.

Note When describing the mass or organ that is enlarged (liver, kidney or spleen), note whether you can get above it, whether it moves with inspiration, whether there is a notch (suggests spleen) or whether it is bimanually ballotable (suggests kidney).

Percussion

- Percuss from the nipple downwards on both sides to locate the upper part of the liver on the right side and the upper part of the spleen on the left side.
- Fluid thrill:
  - Put your left hand on the patient's right flank.
  - Using your right hand, gently flick the skin on the abdominal wall over the left flank using the thumb.
  - If ascites is present, your left hand, which is on the flank, will detect a thrill.
  - Percuss for shifting dullness.
  - Confirm the presence of ascites by percussing from the umbilicus (resonant) to the flanks (stony dull).
  - Mark the level or keep the finger in place at the point where percussion has become stony dull.
  - Ask the patient to roll to their left side. Pause for 30 seconds.
  - If ascites is present, the percussion note where your finger has been placed is now resonant. This is because the fluid has shifted from the right to the left flank.

Auscultation

- Check for:
  - bowel sounds
  - liver bruit
  - renal artery bruit
  - aortic aneurysm

On completion

- Tell the examiner that you would like to complete the examination with a rectal examination, examine the external genitalia and check for ankle oedema.

Examination of the respiratory system

Introduction

- Introduce yourself to the patient and ask for their consent to examine them.
- Ensure that the chest is completely exposed.
- Ensure that the patient is sitting comfortably at 45 degrees.

Inspection

General inspection

- Check around the bedside for cigarettes, oxygen cylinder or inhalers.
- Check the sputum pot.
- Note if the patient is cachectic, short of breath or if there is any obvious asymmetry of the chest wall when viewed from the foot of the bed.
- Listen to the patient breathing with the unaided ear, listening for cough, wheeze, stridor or laboured breathing.
- Note if the expiratory phase is prolonged, as in COPD.
- Assess the respiratory rate to determine if the patient is tachypnoeic.

Hands

- Inspect the hands for:
  - clubbing – found in malignancy, bronchiectasis, empyema, CF and fibrosing alveolitis
  - peripheral cyanosis
  - nicotine staining of fingers
  - purpura from steroid use
  - wasting of the small muscles of the hand
  - fine tremor of the hands due to treatment with β-agonists
  - asterixis – flapping tremor when wrists are dorsiflexed due to carbon dioxide
  - retention – seen in respiratory failure
- Check the pulse to see if it is bounding or tachycardic.

Face

- Inspect the eyes for pallor (suggesting anaemia) or Horner's syndrome.
- Inspect the mouth for pursed-lip breathing.

- Inspect the tongue looking for central cyanosis for COPD or pulmonary fibrosis.

Neck

- Inspect the JVP which is fixed in SVCO and raised in cor pulmonale.
- Inspect for any scars, such as a phrenic nerve crush scar in the supraclavicular fossa.

Chest wall

- Inspect the chest wall for thoracotomy scars and radiotherapy tattoos.
- Assess the shape of the chest wall – barrel shaped in emphysema, pectus carinatum, which can occur following childhood respiratory illness or rickets, or pectus excavatum.
- Observe whether the accessory muscles are being used, as seen in asthma.
- Inspect the movements of the chest wall:
  - asymmetrical movements are seen if there is an underlying pneumothorax, pleural effusion, consolidation or pneumonectomy
  - upwards movement of the chest wall occurs in emphysema

Palpation

Apex beat

- Displacement suggests mediastinal displacement as in collapse, fibrosis, pneumonectomy and pleural effusion.

Neck

- Palpate for cervical and axillary lymphadenopathy, which can be present in carcinoma, tuberculosis and lymphoma.
- Palpate the trachea with the index and ring fingers on either side of the manubrium sternae and the middle finger to locate the trachea.
- Assess for tracheal deviation* and cricoid–suprasternal notch distance, which is decreased in hyperinflation.

*The trachea is deviated to the side of collapse but deviates away from the side of a pleural effusion or mass.

Chest expansion*

- Measure the distance between the thumbs and mid-line in centimetres in the inframammary regions.
- This may be reduced on one side or bilaterally and suggests underlying pathology.

*Assess chest movements posteriorly by sitting the patient forward. Grasp the chest from behind with two hands in the region of T10. Bring the thumbs together, and then ask the patient to breathe in.

We recommend that you perform chest expansion at the front of the chest, followed by percussion and auscultation of the anterior chest wall. Following this, we would recommend continuing to the back, measuring chest expansion and then performing percussion and auscultation.

Percussion*

- Percuss the supraclavicular areas, clavicles and the upper, middle and lower lobes on the anterior chest wall.

*When percussing, it is important to compare the opposite side as you percuss down the chest wall. For example, percuss the left supraclavicular area and then the right supraclavicular area. Percuss the left clavicle and then the right. DO NOT percuss the entire left side and then percuss the right side.

Auscultation

- Auscultate the supraclavicular areas, lower, middle and upper lobes.
- Comment on the breath sounds and added sounds.

Breath sounds

- Vesicular or bronchial
- Normal or reduced

Added sounds

- Wheeze
- Early inspiratory crackles occur in COPD and asthma
- Late inspiratory crackles occur in pulmonary fibrosis
- Early and mid-inspiratory crackles that change when coughing suggest bronchiectasis
- Fine crackles occur in pulmonary fibrosis and pulmonary oedema
- Coarse crackles occur in pneumonia
- Pleural rub
- Perform vocal resonance over all the areas of auscultation. It is reduced in pleural effusion and increased in consolidation

Complete the examination

- Ask the patient to sit forwards and examine the posterior chest wall:
  - chest expansion
  - percussion
  - auscultation
  - vocal resonance

Examination of the locomotor system

Hands

Introduction

- Introduce yourself to the patient and ask for consent to examine them.
- Ensure that the patient is exposed from the hands to the elbow.
- Ensure that the patient is sitting comfortably; place a pillow under the hands.

Look

General inspection of face

- Beaked nose and facial telangiectasia are suggestive of systemic sclerosis
- Heliotrope rash of dermatomyositis
- Cushingoid features due to steroid use for rheumatoid arthritis and SLE

Inspection of the hands

- Inspect the joints:
  - swan neck deformity
  - boutonniere deformity
  - Z deformity of the thumbs
  - ulnar deviation of the fingers
  - swelling of the distal IPJs suggests psoriatic arthropathy
  - swelling of the proximal IPJs and MCPJs suggests rheumatoid arthritis
  - note any surgical scars from carpal tunnel surgery or joint replacement
- Inspect the nails:
  - nail-fold infarcts seen in rheumatoid arthritis, SLE and systemic sclerosis
  - nail pitting, onycholysis, ridging, hyperkeratosis are found in psoriasis
- Inspect the dorsum of the hand:
  - Heberden's nodes occur in osteoarthritis
  - Bouchard's nodes occur in osteoarthritis
  - gouty tophi
  - steroid purpura
  - wasting of small muscles of the hand
  - digital ischaemia as found in systemic sclerosis
  - sclerodactyly and calcified nodules of systemic sclerosis
  - Raynaud's phenomenon is often found in systemic sclerosis and SLE
- Inspect the palms and wrist area:
  - palmar erythema
  - wasting of the thenar or hypothenar eminence
  - thickening of the palmar fascia due to Dupuytren's contracture

Feel

- Ask the patient if they are in pain or have any areas of tenderness.
- Feel the skin, assessing the temperature of both hands.
- Feel for thickening of the palmar fascia due to Dupuytren's contracture.

- Feel the joints for synovitis by gently pressing both sides of the patient's joint with your index finger and thumb of one hand. Press on the middle of the patient's joint with the fingers of your other hand.
- Feel the pulps of the fingers for calcinosis.

Move

- Ask the patient to perform the 'prayer sign', in which the wrists are extended at 90 degrees.
- Ask the patient to flex the wrists at 90 degrees with the dorsal wrist surfaces touching.
- Ask the patient to point the thumb to the ceiling. Push down against it to assess for weakness. This tests the abductor pollicus brevis muscle, which is supplied by the median nerve.
- Ask them to spread their fingers and try to push them together. This tests the dorsal interosseus muscles which are supplied by the ulnar nerve.
- Ask them to hold a piece of paper between their fingers. Try to pull this out. This tests the palmar interosseus muscles which are supplied by the ulnar nerve.

Check function

- Ask the patient to unbutton their shirt or jacket.
- Ask the patient to pick up a set of keys with their fingers.
- Observe how well the patient can write.

Sensation

- Check the little finger to see if there is ulnar nerve involvement.
- Check the index finger and thumb to see if there is median nerve involvement.
- Check the lateral aspect of the base of the thumb to see if there is radial nerve involvement.
- Perform Tinel's sign (tap over the flexor retinaculum to detect median nerve entrapment).
- Check Froment's sign, which is a test for ulnar nerve palsy and specifically tests the action of the adductor pollicis. Ask the patient to hold a piece of paper between the thumb and a flat palm as the paper is pulled away. The patient with an ulnar nerve palsy will flex the thumb to try to maintain a hold on the paper.

Elbows

- Look and feel for rheumatoid nodules, gouty tophi, psoriatic plaques and surgical scars, such as those from ulnar nerve decompression.

Finish

- Offer to examine the other joints or organs which may be affected in rheumatoid arthritis or SLE.

Knees

Introduction

- Introduce yourself to the patient and ask for consent to examine them.
- Ensure that both legs are exposed from the upper thigh to the feet.
- Ensure that the patient is comfortable – ideally he or she should be lying down on a bed.

Look

General inspection

- Note if the patient uses any walking aids.
- Note any psoriatic plaques on elbows, face or knees.
- Note any symmetrical deforming arthropathy of rheumatoid arthritis in the hands.

Inspection of the knees

- Compare both knees and look for:
  - joint effusion
  - joint swelling
  - deformity of the leg
  - wasting of the quadriceps muscle
  - surgical scars from joint replacement

Feel

- Ask the patient if they are in any pain or if there are any areas of tenderness.
- Feel the temperature of the skin overlying the knee and note if it is warm.
- Palpate the popliteal fossa for a mass such as a Baker's cyst.
- While the knee is extended, ask the patient to flex it, placing your hand over the joint and feeling for crepitus.
- Perform the 'patellar tap' test:
  - This tests for a large effusion
  - Press over the suprapatellar bursa with the flat of one hand, squeezing any fluid from it with the index finger and thumb while moving your fingers from the lower part of the quadriceps to the upper part of the patella
  - With the fingers of your other hand, press down on the patella with a quick movement
  - If you feel a 'tap' as the patella hits the lower end of the femur, then an effusion is preset
- Perform the 'bulge test':
  - This tests for a small effusion
  - The suprapatellar bursa is first emptied of fluid by squeezing above the patella with one hand
  - The medial compartment is then emptied by massaging the medial side of the joint with the free hand. This hand is then lifted away and then the lateral side is sharply compressed
  - If the test is positive, a ripple is seen on the flattened, medial surface

Move

- Note whether the patient can passively flex and extend the knee, or if movement is reduced.

Check for stability of the medial collateral ligament
- Ensure that the knee is fully extended.
- Place one hand on the lateral side of the knee and the other hand on the medial side of the ankle.
- Try to push the ankle laterally while pushing the knee medially.
- If there is a significant amount of movement of the knee medially, it suggests laxity of the medial collateral ligament.

Check for stability of the lateral collateral ligament
- Ensure that the knee is fully extended.
- Place one hand on the medial side of the knee and the other on the lateral side of the ankle.
- Try to push the ankle medially while pushing the knee laterally.
- If there is a significant amount of movement of the knee laterally, it suggests laxity of the lateral collateral ligament.

Check for stability of the anterior cruciate ligament
- Flex the knee to 90 degrees.
- Steady the foot by sitting close to it (but not on it).
- Place both your thumbs on the tibial tuberosity.
- Grasp the lower leg and pull it towards you.
- If there is a large amount of movement anteriorly, this suggests laxity of the anterior cruciate ligament.

Check for stability of the posterior cruciate ligament
- Flex the knee to 90 degrees.
- Steady the foot by sitting close to it (but not on it).
- Place both your thumbs on the tibial tuberosity.
- Grasp the lower leg and push it away from you.
- If there is a large amount of movement posteriorly, this suggests laxity of the posterior cruciate ligament.

Feet

Introduction

- Introduce yourself to the patient and ask for consent to examine them.
- Ensure that the patient is comfortable.
- Ensure that the feet are completely exposed.

Look

- Skin rashes
- Scars
- Psoriatic plaques
- Hallux valgus

- Clawing and crowding of the toes
- Check the medial and longitudinal arches of the foot

Feel

- Ask the patient if they are in pain or have any areas of tenderness.
- Check the temperature of the feet and compare both sides.
- Palpate the MTPJ for tenderness.
- Palpate the digits for synovial thickening.
- Palpate the heel for plantar fasciitis.
- Palpate the Achilles tendon for thickening or nodules.

Move

- Assess patient's gait.
- Assess ankle inversion and eversion, dorsiflexion and plantar flexion.

Spine

Introduction

- Introduce yourself to the patient and ask for consent to examine them.
- Ensure that the patient is comfortable.
- Ensure that the spine is completely exposed.

Look

- With the patient standing, observe the posture from behind, assessing for kyphosis and scoliosis.
- Observe the posture from the side, checking for normal lordosis or the characteristic question mark posture of ankylosing spondylitis.
- Examine for any surgical scars.

Feel

- Ask the patient if they are in any pain or discomfort.
- Palpate the spinous processes checking for tenderness.

Move

- Assess spinal movements including forward flexion, lateral flexion and rotation.

Special tests

- Occiput-to-wall test assesses the loss of cervical range of motion. Normally, when the heels and scapulae touch the wall, the occiput touches the wall. In ankylosing spondylitis, the patient is unable to touch the wall with his or her occiput.
- Schober's test detects the amount of lumbar flexion. A mark is made at the level of the posterior superior iliac spine on the vertebral column (approximately at the level of L5). Place one finger 5 cm below this mark and another at 10 cm above the mark. The patient is then asked to touch his or her toes. When the

patient flexes forward, the measured distance should increase by at least 5 cm. However, if the increase in distance between the two fingers on the patient's spine is less than 5 cm, this suggests that mobility of the lumbar spine is reduced.

Examination of the thyroid

Introduction

- Introduce yourself to the patient and ask for consent to examine them.
- Ensure that the neck is adequately exposed.
- Ensure that the patient is in a sitting position and is comfortable.

Inspection

General inspection

- Stand back and have a look at the patient to try to assess whether he or she is hyperthyroid, hypothyroid, euthyroid or has a goitre.
- The patient may be fidgety and restless if hyperthyroid, or the movements may be slow if they are hypothyroid.
- The patient may be slim if hyperthyroid or overweight if hypothyroid.
- Dress may be appropriate for the temperature, suggesting that the patient is euthyroid. If they have several layers on, it may suggest that they are hypothyroid. If they have thin clothing, it may suggest that they are hyperthyroid.

Hands

- Check for tremor by asking the patient to outstretch their hands. If tremor is not visible, place a piece of paper on the outstretched hands. It will shake if there is a fine tremor.
- Check for hot, sweaty palms and palmar erythema.
- Check for thyroid acropachy.
- Check the pulse for tachycardia or AF (hyperthyroidism) or bradycardia (hypothyroidism).

Neck

- Goitre – if you see a goitre ask the patient to take a sip of water and then observe them swallowing. If a goitre is present, the mass will move up.
- Ask the patient to stick the tongue out – if the mass moves up when doing this, the patient has a thyroglossal cyst.
- Check for surgical scars from previous thyroidectomy.
- Check for cervical lymphadenopathy.

Face

- Proptosis – best seen from above and behind the patient
- Exophthalmos – lower sclera is visible
- Lid retraction – upper sclera is visible

- Lid lag – move your finger quickly downwards and ask the patient to follow it while fixing their forehead with your other hand
- Chemosis
- Ophthalmoplegia
- Loss of outer third of the eyebrows

Legs

- Look for pre-tibial myxoedema on the shins.
- Check the ankle reflexes, which are delayed in hypothyroidism.

Palpation

- Ask the patient if they have any tenderness or pain in the neck.
- Palpate the thyroid gland from behind the patient:
  - size
  - tenderness suggests thyroiditis
  - mobility – ask the patient to swallow some water to determine if the goitre is mobile; if it is fixed, this may suggest an invasive thyroid carcinoma
  - consistency – solitary nodule, multiple nodules, diffusely swollen
  - texture – smooth in goitres, hard or knobbly if carcinoma
- Palpate for cervical lymphadenopathy.
- Check for tracheal deviation.
- Check for Pemberton's sign. Ask the patient to raise their arms above their head. If they have a retrosternal goitre, they may develop giddiness, suffusion of the face or syncope.

Percussion

- Percuss over the upper sternum to assess for a retrosternal goitre.

Auscultation

- Listen over the thyroid gland for a bruit.

On completion

- Tell the examiner that you would investigate this patient with TFTs.

CHAPTER 3 FURTHER READING

Adams HP Jr, del Zoppo G, Alberts MJ, *et al.* Guidelines for the early management of adults with ischemic stroke. *Stroke* 2007; 38: 1655–711.

Bloom S, Webster G, Marks D. *Oxford Handbook of Gastroenterolgy and Hepatology.* Oxford, UK: Oxford University Press, 2006.

British Thoracic Society and Scottish Intercollegiate Guidelines Network. *British Guideline on the Management of Asthma.* London: BTS, 2009. www.brit-thoracic.org.uk/Portals/0/Guidelines/AsthmaGuidelines/qrg101%20revised%202009.pdf (accessed 14 February 2012).

Chapman S, Robinson G, Stradling J, West S. *Oxford Handbook of Respiratory Medicine.* Oxford, UK: Oxford University Press, 2009.

Collier J, Longmore M, Turmezei T, Mafi A. *Oxford Handbook of Clinical Specialties*, 8th edition. Oxford, UK: Oxford University Press, 2009.

Douglas G, Nicol F, Robertson C (eds). *Macleod's Clinical Examination.* London: Churchill Livingstone, 2009.

European Heart Rhythm Association; European Association for Cardio-Thoracic Surgery, Camm AJ, *et al.* Guidelines for the management of atrial fibrillation: the Task Force for the Management of Atrial Fibrillation of the European Society of Cardiology (ESC). *European Heart Journal* 2010; 31: 2369–429.

Ewing JA. Detecting alcoholisim. The CAGE questionnaire. *Journal of the American Medical Association* 1984; 252: 1905–7.

Hakim A, Clunie G, Haq I. *Oxford Handbook of Rheumatology*, 2nd edition. Oxford, UK: Oxford University Press, 2006.

Kumar P, Clark ML (eds). *Kumar and Clark's Clinical Medicine*, 7th edition. Philadelphia: Saunders Elsevier, 2009.

Longmore M, Wilkinson I, Davidson E, Foulkes A, Mafi A. *Oxford Handbook of Clinical Medicine*, 8th edition. Oxford, UK: Oxford University Press, 2010.

National Institute for Clinical Excellence. Multiple sclerosis. *Management of multiple sclerosis in primary and secondary care*, NICE guideline CG8. London: NICE, 2003. www.nice.org.uk/CG8 (accessed 14 February 2012).

National Institute for Health and Clinical Excellence. *Prophylaxis against infective endocarditis*, NICE guideline CG064. London: NICE, 2008. www.guidance.nice.org.uk/CG064 (accessed 14 February 2012).

National Institute for Health and Clinical Excellence. *Type 2 diabetes: newer agents for blood glucose control in type 2 diabetes*, NICE guideline CG66. London: NICE, 2008. www.guidance.nice.org.uk/CG66 (accessed 14 February 2012).

National Institute for Health and Clinical Excellence. *Chronic heart failure. Management of chronic heart failure in adults in primary and secondary care*, NICE guideline CG108. London: NICE, 2010. www.guidance.nice.org.uk/CG108 (accessed 14 February 2012).

National Institute for Health and Clinical Excellence (2010) *Chronic obstructive pulmonary disease (updated)*, NICE guideline CG101. London: NICE. http://guidance.nice.org.uk/CG101 (accessed 14 February 2012).

Ryder B, Mir A, Freeman A. *An Aid to the MRCP Paces. Volume 1: Stations 1, 3 and 5*, 3rd edition. Chichester: Wiley-Blackwell, 2003.

Souhami RL, Moxham J (eds). *Textbook of Medicine*, 3rd edition. London: Churchill Livingstone, 1997.